LOWER LDL CHOLESTEROL NATURALLY WITH FOOD

Simple Ways to Add Proven LDL Reducers to Your Everyday Routine

MICHAEL GREGER, M.D., FACLM

New York Times Bestselling Author of *How Not to Die, How Not to Diet,* and *How Not to Age*

Founder of NutritionFacts.org

with Kristine Dennis, PhD, MPH

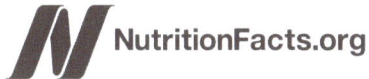

Also by Michael Greger, M.D., FACLM

How Not to Die

The How Not to Die Cookbook

How Not to Diet

The How Not to Diet Cookbook

How to Survive a Pandemic

How Not to Age

The How Not to Age Cookbook

This book contains the opinions and ideas of its authors. It is intended to provide helpful general information on the subjects that it addresses. It is not in any way a substitute for the advice of the reader's own physician(s) or other medical professionals based on the reader's own individual conditions, symptoms, or concerns. If the reader needs personal medical, health, dietary, exercise, or other assistance or advice, the reader should consult a competent physician and/or other qualified health care professionals. The authors and publisher specifically disclaim all responsibility for injury, damage, or loss that the reader may incur as a direct or indirect consequence of following any directions or suggestions given in the book or participating in any programs described in the book.

LOWER LDL CHOLESTEROL NATURALLY WITH FOOD. Copyright © 2025 by NutritionFacts.org. All rights reserved. Printed in the United States of America. For information, address NutritionFacts.org, P.O. Box 11400, Takoma Park, MD 20913.

ISBN 979-8-9916605-4-9 (paperback)
ISBN 979-8-9916605-5-6 (e-book)

The Library of Congress Cataloging-in-Publication Data is available upon request.

LCCN: 2025916570

First paperback edition, October 2025

Cover design, figures, and charts by Robert King Design. Cover art by Kat Farrell, NutritionFacts.org. Interior by Typeflow.

CONTENTS

INTRODUCTION	1
STATINS	3
Recommendation Criteria	3
How Effective Are Statins?	5
How Much Benefit Do Patients Expect?	5
Fewer Heart Attacks, but More Diabetes	6
The Side Effects	8
Painfully Overlooked	8
1 in 1,000 or 1 in 10?	9
Tired Truth	9
Dietary Deterrence of Dementia and Death	10
Your Brain on Statins	11
How Cholesterol-Lowering Medications Work	11
Dr. Endo Broke the Mold	12
Which Statin Is the Best?	13

THE PORTFOLIO DIET — 15

Avoiding the Three Things That
Raise LDL Cholesterol — 15

    Trans Fat — 16

    Saturated Fat — 17

    Dietary Cholesterol — 17

Consuming the Four Factors That
Lower LDL Cholesterol — 17

The Portfolio Diet vs. Statins — 18

But Fortified Margarine? — 18

Fiber and Phytosterols Flush Cholesterol — 19

Where Are Plant Sterols Found? — 20

Plant Sterols Safety — 22

    Can Plant Sterols Also Take on Our Second Leading Killer? — 22

    Interference with Fat-Soluble Vitamin Absorption — 23

    Phytosterol Oxidation Products — 23

    Red Blood Cell Fragility? — 24

    Cautionary Tale from Phytosterolemia? — 24

Do Plant Sterols Actually Prevent Heart Attacks? — 25

The Best Dosing of Plant Sterols — 26

The Best Source of Plant Sterols — 27

Cholesterol-Lowering Supplements to Avoid — 28

    No to Policosanol — 28

    No to Red Yeast Rice — 29

Cholesterol-Lowering Supplements to Consider	31
Psyllium Husk	31
Bergamot	31
Artichoke	33
Barberries for Berberine	33
Supplements vs. Statins	35
Foods That Lower Cholesterol	37
Nuts	38
Beans	39
Viscous Fiber and Plant Sterols	39
Barberries and Artichoke Hearts	40
Apples	40
Flaxseeds	40
Herbs and Spices	41
PUTTING IT ALL INTO PRACTICE	**45**
Dr. Greger's Portfolio Plus Powder	46
Starting in Neutral Territory	47
Next, Nasty	50
Lastly, Tasty	51
CONCLUSION	**53**
NOTES	**57**
INDEX	**83**

INTRODUCTION

LDL cholesterol, also known as "bad" cholesterol, is "unequivocally recognized as the principal driving force" in the development of atherosclerotic cardiovascular disease,[1] our leading cause of death.[2] Guidelines have shifted to lower and lower LDL cholesterol targets as more and more clinical trials have demonstrated that lower is better.[3] They started with an LDL goal of 130 mg/dL* in the 1980s and went down to 100 mg/dL in the 1990s, then further still to 70 mg/dL in the 2000s for those at really high risk, and, over the last decade, even lower to 55, 40, or even 30 mg/dL.[4] These more recent targets may actually be closer to what is normal, naturally speaking, for our species. Even after we learned to use tools to hunt, normal LDL was around 50 to 70 mg/dL, but today, the average LDL in the Western world is more like 120 mg/dL.[5] No wonder heart disease is the leading cause of death in men and women.

Recently, guidelines have begun entirely scrapping targets in favor of pushing for LDL levels to be "as low as possible,"[6] given the realization that the lower, the better.[7] Indeed, no threshold seems to exist below which further LDL-lowering therapy does not further reduce risk of major cardiovascular "events" like heart attacks, strokes, or death. In fact, the reduction in risk appears to be independent of the starting LDL cholesterol. Even those individuals who start out with LDL under 80 mg/dL get about the same relative reduction in risk.[8]

---

* To convert mg/dL (used in the United States) to mmol/L (used elsewhere), divide by 38.67. For example, 130 mg/dL ÷ 38.67 = 3.36 mmol/L.

So, even with an LDL less than 100 mg/dL that your doctor may consider "normal,"[9] it is considered of "utmost importance" to lower it further,[10] even if other heart disease risk factors are considered optimal.[11] In that case, why aren't statins prescribed for everyone?[12] Because there are risks of side effects (in addition to the burden of taking a pill every day for the rest of our life).[13] That's why these drugs are only recommended for those at relatively high risk of having a heart attack for whom the pros of cholesterol-lowering outweigh the cons of taking the drug.[14] Nearly all may benefit in some way from adding a statin, but the question is *at what cost?*

So, we know that "lower is better for longer" when it comes to LDL and "the earlier the better," and the primary reason drugs aren't more frequently prescribed is because of their drawbacks.[15] What if there were safe, simple, side-effect-free solutions to lowering our cholesterol? For example, what if we could lower our LDL by eating specific types of healthy foods every day? If that were the case, then regardless of whether we're on drugs, wouldn't we want to utilize every safe, no-downside strategy there is to get our LDL as low as possible? That's what this book is all about.

STATINS

According to the latest cholesterol clinical practice guidelines from the American Heart Association and the American College of Cardiology, the number one take-home message is to lead a lifelong heart-healthy lifestyle. Dietary modification in particular is considered the cornerstone of LDL lowering,[16] but at what point are drugs also recommended? If you have diagnosed heart disease, like if you've already had a heart attack and are trying to prevent another, then drugs are considered non-negotiable.[17] But what about in the context of *primary* prevention, meaning preventing that first heart attack? At what point do the benefits outweigh the risks?

Recommendation Criteria

With an LDL of 190 mg/dL or more, it's recommended to go straight to statins. Don't pass *Go*, don't collect $200. Statins are also automatically recommended for those aged 40 to 75 years with diabetes who have an LDL of even 70 mg/dL. For individuals without known cardiovascular disease or diabetes and an LDL between 70 and 190 mg/dL, then statins are generally recommended if the risk of having a cardiovascular event, like a heart attack or stroke, is 7.5% or more over the next ten years.[18]

Even a ten-year risk as low as 5% may merit a statin recommendation, if certain "risk-enhancing factors" are present, such as a family history of early cardiovascular disease, chronic kidney disease, premature menopause, inflammatory diseases such as rheumatoid arthritis, South Asian ancestry, persistently elevated triglycerides (≥ 175 mg/dL or 1.98 mmol/L), high C-reactive protein (hs-CRP ≥ 2.0 mg/L), or high Lp(a) (≥ 50 mg/dL or 125 nmol/L). As one's ten-year risk approaches 20%, immediate statin initiation is recommended to cut LDL levels at least in half. In the intermediate risk range between 7.5% and 20%, statins are also recommended. If you're still on the fence, a coronary calcium scan imaging test can be done to help you decide. Delaying statin initiation is considered reasonable in that intermediate risk range if your coronary calcium scan is zero and you lack any risk-enhancing factors.[19]

How do you determine your ten-year risk? There are a variety of risk calculators available online. My favorite is u-prevent.com. It's free and endorsed by the European Society of Cardiology.* Not only does it give you a ten-year risk estimate, as well as a lifetime risk estimate, but it also estimates *when* the event may occur.[20] Best of all, you can toggle between various treatment options to see what may happen to your risk if you follow them. For instance, you can learn the effect on your predicted risk if you stop smoking, increase your step count, or start a statin.[21]

According to the calculator, as an example, if a 60-year-old smoking woman with an LDL of 140 mg/dL does nothing, her ten-year year risk of suffering a cardiovascular event may be 8.6%. Since that is greater than 7.5%, she would likely obtain a net benefit from starting a statin. Ultimately, though, it's her decision. A review on communicating statin evidence to patients concluded:

> [W]hether or not the overall benefit-harm balance justifies the use of a medication for an individual patient cannot be determined by a guidelines committee, a health care system, or even the attending physician. Instead, it is the individual patient who has a fundamental right to decide whether or not taking a drug is worthwhile.[22]

So, allow me to go through the pros and cons so you can decide for yourself.

---

* Note that to use u-prevent.com, you have to check a box saying that you're a health professional (presumably for liability reasons). If you're not comfortable doing so, you can use the American Heart Association's simplified PREVENT calculator at see.nf/prevent.

How Effective Are Statins?

Physicians have been criticized for paternalistically misleading patients about the risks and benefits of statins.[23] Surveys show most patients expect greater benefit from drugs such as statins than the actual benefit they provide, which creates tension between a patient's right to know and the likely reduction in the chance they would agree to take a drug if they knew how little benefit it offered.[24] On a population-scale, that would be devastating. Statins likely prevent tens of thousands of deaths a year in the United States alone, for example. If patients were routinely told the truth as to how little benefit they could expect on an individual level, as many as 75% of patients might stop treatment. So, unless everyone is kept in the dark, 30,000 people could die.[25] What should doctors do?

I agree with those who believe we have to tell our patients the truth even if it means someone decides not to take the drug and potentially dies as a result. It's their body, their choice.[26] (I wish those informed consent enthusiasts would extend such sentiment to telling patients about the beneficial role a healthy diet can play![27])

Are you in the 25% who would take statins even knowing the full picture? Let's find out.

How Much Benefit Do Patients Expect?

Prescription drug ads are everywhere—that is, if you live in the United States or New Zealand, the only two "major" countries in which they aren't illegal.[28] One such ad of the statin drug Lipitor claims it reduces the risk of heart attack by about a third. The fine print at the bottom reads: "That means in a large clinical study, 3% of patients taking a sugar pill had a heart attack compared to 2% of patients taking Lipitor."[29] Going from 3% down to 2% is indeed a drop by a third in *relative risk*, but the drop in *absolute risk* is only 1%, which sounds less impressive.

The emphasis on relative risk to embellish the benefit is common even within the medical literature, which is no surprise since journal articles are often written by drug manufacturers themselves.[30] Now, the drop in heart attacks from 3% to 2% on Lipitor was over a period of only about three years. These are drugs to be taken over a lifetime, so their benefits accrue.[31] Over four or five years on a statin, for instance, the absolute risk reduction might go up to 1.3%, but you can see why many patients may still not be very moved.[32] A systematic review of patient preferences found that even in studies where people were asked to imagine an idealized tablet free of side effects, more than a third stated they would not consider taking it unless it reduced their five-year absolute risk by at least 5%.[33]

Researchers found that only about 50% of people would apparently consider taking preventive medications that prolonged their life by less than eight months.[34] The average expected longevity benefit from statins ranges from a few months to a few years, depending on risk. To offset the "inconvenience of having to take a daily tablet," about a third of patients would settle for just three more months, whereas about one in ten individuals said they wouldn't take pills even if they got to live an extra ten years or more.[35] That's mind-boggling to me, but that's why it's such a personal decision. People are all over the place in terms of what they're willing to accept. Your doctor, however, may not care.

Physicians were presented with the case of a man with a 7% to 10% risk of dying from cardiovascular disease over the next decade who explicitly said he would only take a statin if it would increase his lifespan by a certain amount. Some doctors were told the patient required at least eight years of life, and others were told he asked for only a matter of months, which is what would actually be gained, on average, in real life. Nevertheless, 83% of the doctors said they would recommend the drug to the patient who unrealistically demanded eight years of life, which is almost the exact percentage recommended by the doctors who were told he wanted only a matter of months. In other words, the doctors were "insensitive to patient preferences regarding survival gain."[36]

Fewer Heart Attacks, but More Diabetes

For primary prevention, trying to prevent our first heart attack, no overall survival benefits have been found for statins.[37] Indeed, only one in eight such studies has shown that statins extend people's lifespan.[38] However, that may be because the studies lasted only a few years, and for low-risk populations, the risk of dying from cardiovascular disease in that time period may be just a few percent anyway. Such trials do show fewer events—fewer heart attacks and strokes—so, on a public health scale, one could argue it makes sense not to wait for individuals to have a heart attack before starting them on cholesterol-lowering drugs.[39]

Critics concede this would be reasonable "if statins had these benefits without side effects," but statins increase the risk of developing diabetes. They suggest these drugs may give as many people diabetes as it prevents them from having a heart attack or stroke.[40] The statistic they cite, though, is from a combination of primary and secondary prevention trials.

In primary prevention trials, there is no increased diabetes risk. That is seen only in secondary prevention trials in which people are trying to prevent their *second* heart attack, for instance.[41] This might be due to the higher doses of statins being used in secondary prevention, as more intensive statin therapy is associated with a greater increased risk of new-onset diabetes compared with more moderate doses.[42] Of course, intensive therapy also offers more benefits in terms of cardiovascular protection.[43] The diabetes risk from statins in secondary prevention trials might also be because the population is at a higher risk of diabetes in general.[44]

If the primary prevention trials are separated by the populations who have low or high rates of diabetes regardless of the drug, statins only appear to increase risk among those with a high baseline rate.[45] Again, this difference between primary versus secondary prevention could be a consequence of running short-term trials in low-risk populations.[46] The big benefit (e.g., preventing death) may not show up, but the big downside (e.g., causing diabetes) may not show up either. However, even in the trials that do show increased diabetes, the risk of getting diabetes would likely be "vastly offset by the cardiovascular protection offered from statin therapy."[47] Of course, a healthy diet may reduce the risk of both concurrently, but before we get to food, what about the other side effects of statins? Increased diabetes risk isn't the only one. What about risks to our muscles, liver, kidney, and brain?

The Side Effects

The primary reason people stop taking statins or refuse to take them altogether seems to be concern about their side effects.[48]

As I mentioned, statins are considered mandatory for secondary prevention for those with known cardiovascular disease,[49] but their use for primary prevention, trying to prevent a first heart attack or stroke, is more of a gray area. One hundred adults aged 50 to 75 without known cardiovascular disease would have to be treated with a statin for two and a half years to prevent a single major adverse cardiovascular event.[50] Put another way, if 10,000 such people were treated for a year, 19 heart attacks, 9 strokes, and 8 cardiovascular deaths would be prevented.[51] That's the upside.

The downside? Of those 10,000 patients, the statins would be expected to cause 15 more cases of muscle issues, 8 more cases of liver dysfunction, 12 more cases of kidney dysfunction, and 14 more eye conditions. So, the likelihood of suffering a major side effect is approximately the same as obtaining a major benefit, but a perk like preventing a heart attack or death is much more important than avoiding a case of blurred vision. This is why some reviewers conclude that "the cardiovascular benefits of statins outweigh adverse effects in primary prevention."[52] But, wait. There were only 15 cases of muscle problems out of 10,000 people treated?

Painfully Overlooked

The rate of major muscle side effects was based on clinical trials that found approximately 1 in 1,000 users develops serious muscle disease over a ten-year period.[53] Cases of muscle weakness or muscle breakdown are hard to miss, whereas the incidence of statin-induced muscle aches and pains is far more contentious.[54] Such randomized controlled trials may seriously underestimate adverse effects like muscle pain, since industry-sponsored trials include run-in periods before the study even starts to exclude people who can't tolerate the drugs.[55] It's no wonder we see such low rates in the actual trials since all those individuals who suffered never went on to participate in them.

Observational studies out in the real world, on the other hand, don't find muscle symptoms in 1 in 1,000 individuals, but rather 1 in 10 or even 1 in 5. That's a rate of 100 to 200 times higher than noted in the trials.[56]

Some have attributed the difference in rates between observational and experimental studies to the *nocebo effect*, where patients experience side effects they are expecting, but it's really all in their heads.[57] Or it could be because, in nearly all the trials, participants were never asked about muscle side effects[58] since there's an incentive not to ask in studies funded by the drug manufacturers.[59] And even when participants were asked, industry-sponsored trials are known to underreport to sweep adverse effects under the rug. What's more, statin trials have often excluded patients with a history of muscle problems, who may be in the population most at risk.[60] So, is it primarily in their heads or in their muscles?

1 in 1,000 or 1 in 10?

To find out what proportion of people have muscle aches caused by the drugs, researchers randomized patients who claimed to be statin-intolerant with actual statins or identical-looking placebos. Could they tell the difference? Only a third to a half of patients consistently reported muscle pain on statins, but not on placebo. So, yes, perhaps most who believe statins are causing their muscle pains are mistaken, but a significant proportion really are suffering because of these drugs.[61] The European Atherosclerosis Society estimates the overall risk of developing statin-related muscle symptoms to be anywhere from 1 in 14 to nearly 1 in 3 people.[62]

Tired Truth

Most trials also do not systematically ask about other potential adverse effects, like fatigue, even though fatigue is among the most commonly reported problems by patients on statins.[63] In a non-industry-funded trial on the effects of statins on energy and fatigue with exertion, compared to placebo, four out of ten women treated with Zocor (simvastatin) cited worsening in either energy levels or exertional fatigue. Women appeared to be more adversely affected,[64] which helps explain why statin-induced fatigue had been underestimated, since, until more recently, statin trials were overwhelmingly gender-biased towards men,[65] even though heart disease is also the leading killer of women.

Dietary Deterrence of Dementia and Death

In 2024, Dr. Dean Ornish published a landmark study showing that a whole food, plant-based diet and other healthy lifestyle behaviors seemed to reverse the progression of early-stage Alzheimer's disease, following his previous work showing that a similar plant-based diet and lifestyle could reverse the progression of heart disease.[66] But it doesn't have to be all or nothing.

In the Lyon Diet Heart Study, heart attack survivors were randomized either to advice to eat a more Mediterranean-style diet rich in plant-based omega-3s or to continue to eat whatever their doctors instructed. The Mediterranean dietary advice group ended up eating more bread and fruit, and less ham, sausage, other meat, butter, and cream. Although they didn't significantly change their fish consumption, they did eat more of a butter-less spread that had been provided, enriched with plant-based omega-3s, like the kind found in flaxseeds and walnuts. The results? Over the next five years, only about 5% of those in the dietary advice group suffered a fatal or nonfatal heart attack, compared to more than 20% of the individuals in the control group.[67]

The first chair of Harvard's Department of Preventive Medicine[68] editorialized:

> At a time when health professionals, the pharmaceutical industries, and the research funding and regulatory agencies are almost totally focused on lowering plasma cholesterol levels by drugs, it is heartening to see a well-conducted study finding that relatively simple dietary changes achieved greater reductions in risk of all-cause and coronary heart disease mortality...than any of the cholesterol-lowering studies to date.[69]

Despite the striking findings—a 70% reduction in the risk of premature death from simply eating more plant foods and less meat and dairy—few cardiologists may even be aware of the study, even though it was published in one of the most prestigious medical journals in the world.[70]

Your Brain on Statins

In 2012, the U.S. Food and Drug Administration (FDA) issued a new warning for the labeling of statin drugs regarding potential adverse effects on cognition, including memory loss and confusion.[71] That was based on earlier studies,[72,73] but, thankfully, more recent evidence does not strongly support a link between statins and cognitive impairment.[74] By 2015, a systematic review concluded that statin therapy does not appear to be associated with cognitive impairment, though that was based on clinical trials beset by the same limitations listed above.[75]

What about statin use and dementia risk? Dozens of studies involving a total of more than seven million patients found that the use of statins was linked to *lower* risks of dementias, such as Alzheimer's disease.[76] This could be due to the part cholesterol plays in the development of dementia. Cholesterol is now universally recognized to be a risk factor for Alzheimer's,[77] helping to explain the role of the "Alzheimer's gene" *APOE*, which is the major cholesterol carrier within the brain.[78] But it could also be due to muddling factors like "healthy user bias," where people who diligently take statins may also engage in other health-promoting behaviors, and it's those behaviors that reduce the risk, rather than the drugs themselves.[79]

How Cholesterol-Lowering Medications Work

To understand how different foods can lower LDL through different mechanisms and thereby potentially have additive effects, we first have to understand the pathways of cholesterol production, absorption, and excretion.

No fewer than 13 Nobel Prizes have been awarded to scientists researching cholesterol,[80] culminating in a constellation of new cholesterol-lowering compounds.[81] Our liver can make cholesterol from scratch through a long series of reactions, which can then be packaged and end up as LDL in our bloodstream to deliver cholesterol throughout our body. We don't want to have too much, as it can lodge in our artery walls, become oxidized, and trigger inflammation that can lead to atherosclerotic plaque and kill us. To prevent this from happening, our liver has LDL receptors that pull LDL from the blood and dispose of cholesterol through our bile by dumping it into our digestive tract, presuming that dietary fiber will trap and ultimately flush it away. If the cholesterol doesn't get trapped, however, it can be reabsorbed and repackaged as LDL, then re-enter our bloodstream. The same absorption happens when we *eat* cholesterol. However, saturated fat is the most important dietary determinant of cholesterol because it reduces the number of liver receptors that remove LDL, so more LDL stays in our blood.[82]

PCSK9 can also reduce our LDL-clearing capacity. It's a protein our liver makes that targets LDL receptors for destruction. In my book *How Not to Age*, I discuss longevity syndromes where some individuals have a faulty PCSK9 gene, which fortuitously leads to more LDL liver receptors and a 90% drop in heart disease risk.[83] This leads to the same kind of boosting of LDL-clearing receptors we get by cutting down on dietary saturated fat intake, regardless of our genetics.[84]

Where do drugs come in? We can cut down on cholesterol production in the first place by blocking its formation with statins or a newer drug called bempedoic acid, blocking the absorption and reabsorption of cholesterol with a drug called ezetimibe, or blocking the production (inclisiran) or the activity (evolocumab and alirocumab) of PCSK9.

In the United States, most of the PCSK9 inhibitors cost about $6,000 annually, with inclisiran closer to $10,000 for the first year. A combination of bempedoic acid and ezetimibe is about $5,000 annually, whereas statins are typically about $50 a year out of pocket or free with insurance.[85] There are two long-acting statins, atorvastatin and rosuvastatin, which can even be taken every other day and cut the cost in half.[86] You can see why statins are the first-line treatment and have been for nearly 40 years.

Dr. Endo Broke the Mold

We recently lost Dr. Akira Endo, who discovered the first statin.[87]

> Microbes are constantly at war with each other. We look to fungi for compounds like penicillin that kill bacteria and to bacteria to find antifungal drugs. Since some microbes rely on cholesterol-like sterols, Dr. Endo was hoping he'd find some other microbe that produced an anti-sterol production compound. After years looking at approximately 6,000 different microbes,[88] in 1972, he came across a blue-green mold that produced something that worked.[89] If he had given up after 5,999 attempts, then millions more people may have died prematurely in the ensuing decades.

Which Statin Is the Best?

If we are going to start a statin, which should we choose? There are currently seven on the market, lowering LDL levels from about 20% to 60% based on brand and dose.[90] In terms of comparative effectiveness and safety for primary prevention, atorvastatin and rosuvastatin have been found to be most effective in reducing cardiovascular disease events, while atorvastatin appears to have the best safety profile.[91] No wonder atorvastatin became the best-selling drug of all time, bringing in more than a hundred billion dollars as Lipitor before it went off patent in 2011.[92]

THE PORTFOLIO DIET

Of the "top ten take-home messages" for the primary prevention of cardiovascular disease from the American College of Cardiology and the American Heart Association, statins come in at number nine. Cholesterol-lowering statin drugs are considered the first-choice drug treatment for preventing heart disease in those with sufficiently elevated LDL cholesterol,[93] though side effects, like muscle pain or weakness, may impact up to a quarter of users.[94] The number one take-home message? "The most important way to prevent atherosclerotic vascular disease," the number one killer of men and women, "heart failure, and atrial fibrillation is to promote a healthy lifestyle throughout life."[95] This is the case regardless of whether or not you and your doctor decide you should start to take drugs.

Enter the Portfolio Diet for the "maximal reduction" of LDL cholesterol with diet.[96]

Avoiding the Three Things That Raise LDL Cholesterol

There are three main factors in our diet that raise LDL cholesterol: trans fat, saturated fat, and dietary cholesterol.[97] Tolerable upper intake levels could not be set for these components, since any intake above zero increases LDL cholesterol concentration and, as such, increases risk of heart disease. So, trans fat, saturated fat, and cholesterol intake should be as low as possible,[98] which means minimizing consumption of meat, dairy, eggs, and junk.[99]

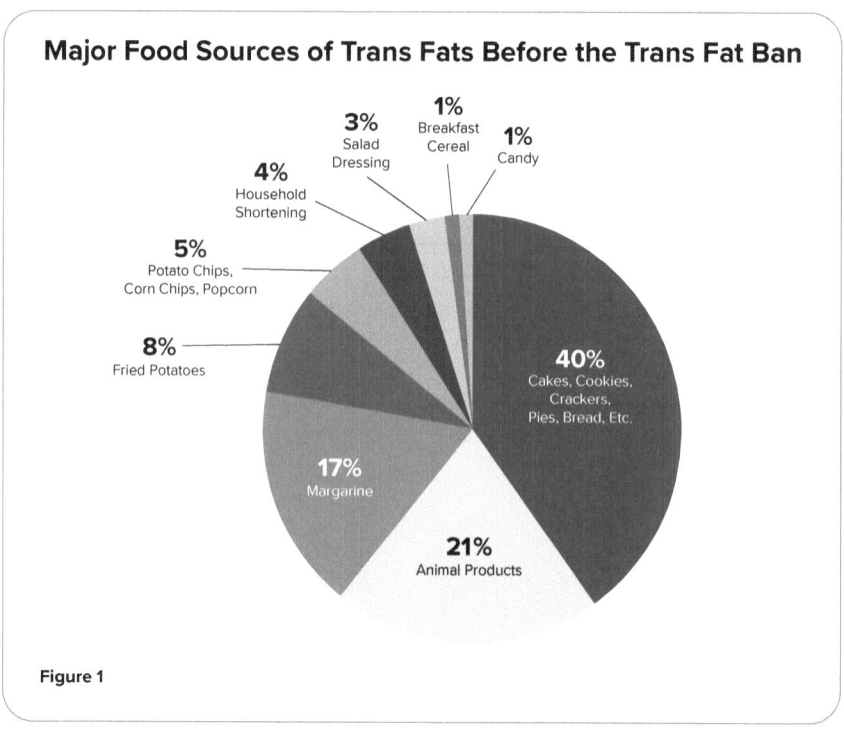

Figure 1

Trans Fat

Figure 1 shows what used to be the major food sources of trans fat for American adults[100] before industrially-produced trans fats in the form of partially hydrogenated oils were removed from the U.S. food supply.[101] However, when it comes to raising LDL, trans fats formed naturally in animals and ending up in meat and dairy may be even worse.[102] Now that trans fats are no longer allowed to be added to processed foods, animal products are the only remaining major source of trans fat in the American diet.[103]

If trans fats are found naturally in meat and dairy and the only safe intake of trans fats is zero, why don't the powers that be more explicitly recommend eating plant-based? As I noted in *How Not to Die*, the director of Harvard's Cardiovascular Epidemiology Program famously explained: "We can't tell people to stop eating all meat and all dairy products…Well, we could tell people to become vegetarians…If we were truly basing this only on science, we would, but it is a bit extreme."[104] We certainly wouldn't want scientists to base anything on science!

Saturated Fat

The leading sources of cholesterol-raising saturated fat in the American diet are dairy (particularly cheese), meat (particularly chicken), and desserts like cookies, cakes, and donuts.[105] Beef tends to have more saturated fat than chicken, but we eat so much more poultry than red meat. However, randomized controlled trials show that switching from beef to chicken or fish fails to lower LDL.[106]

Dietary Cholesterol

Online, some bloggers parrot the egg industry's talking point[107] that the 2015 U.S. Dietary Guidelines *removed* the dietary cholesterol limit, whereas if anyone bothered to *read* the actual guidelines, they'd see that the Guidelines in reality *strengthened* its recommendation by telling Americans to "eat as little dietary cholesterol as possible,"[108] as recommended by the Institute of Medicine, the most prestigious medical body in the United States. This advice was reiterated in the 2020–2025 dietary guidelines: "The National Academies [of Science] recommends that dietary cholesterol consumption to be as low as possible."[109] While eggs are the most concentrated source of cholesterol gram-for-gram, the greatest contribution in the American diet is meat, including poultry and fish.[110]

Consuming the Four Factors That Lower LDL Cholesterol

It follows that those eating more plant-based tend to have lower LDL. In fact, the average LDL for those eating strictly plant-based is as low as 70 mg/dL. Compared to the general public's, that's an excellent number, but, as discussed, there is no safe cut off.[111] It bears repeating: When it comes to our LDL cholesterol, the lower, for longer, the better—even if we're starting out at relatively low risk.[112] So, avoidance alone is not enough. That's where the Portfolio Diet can come in.[113]

Eating a healthy plant-based diet subtracts all the major foods that increase our LDL cholesterol. The Portfolio Diet is plant-based with a bonus—a portfolio of foods we can *add* to our diet to actively pull cholesterol out of our system:[114]

- **Nuts.** Eat 1½ ounces of nuts a day.
- **Plant protein.** Emphasize legumes, including soy, other beans, split peas, chickpeas, or lentils.
- **Viscous fiber.** Emphasize foods with lots of sticky fiber, like oats, okra, eggplant, barley, and flaxmeal.
- **Plant sterols.** With meals, eat a total of 2 grams of plant sterols each day.

The Portfolio Diet vs. Statins

Researchers tested the Portfolio Diet head-to-head against statin treatment plus a very low saturated fat diet in a four-week, randomized, controlled trial among people with high cholesterol. Incredibly, those in the Portfolio group had a nearly 30% drop in LDL cholesterol, similar to the 33% drop observed in the statins plus low saturated fat group. Eating plant-based and emphasizing the addition of four dietary components that are each likely to independently contribute 4% to 7% to overall cholesterol reduction resulted in a diet that lowered LDL cholesterol with drug-like potency—without any drugs.[115]

A systematic review and meta-analysis of controlled trials of the Portfolio Diet showed consistent LDL-lowering benefits, about a 17% drop in LDL beyond that achieved by the typical (National Cholesterol Education Program) cholesterol-lowering diet, along with reductions in systemic inflammation and an estimated 13% decrease in ten-year heart disease risk.[116] Note that these results were not from individuals who actually went on the Portfolio Diet, but rather those merely *instructed* to eat that way. Just two educational sessions over six months telling people to adopt the eating pattern can have a significant effect.[117]

But Fortified Margarine?

Most of the Portfolio Diet's components are familiar, foods like oatmeal, beans, and nuts. However, the source of plant sterols used in many clinical trials was plant-sterol-fortified margarine.[118] It's been available commercially under such brands as Benecol and Promise Activ, formerly known as Take Control. These products have added plant sterols, but they're also ultra-processed nightmares full of salt, saturated fat, and artificial flavors.[119,120]

If one insists on using some sort of buttery spread, these would be better than *non*-fortified margarine or butter, but that seems like a strange way to try to prevent heart disease.

Plant sterols, also known as *phytosterols*, are naturally concentrated in sesame seeds and wheat germ,[121] and found in a variety of nuts, grains, and legumes.[122] But to reach the recommended 2 or 3 grams a day, one would probably need to use plant-sterol-fortified foods or supplements.

So, should we all be taking plant sterol supplements? Any other cholesterol-lowering supplements that might be worth considering? And what about expanding our portfolio? Are there any other foods that have been shown to lower cholesterol? One could imagine developing a Portfolio *Plus* Diet with as many different cholesterol-lowering foods, herbs, and spices as possible. That's exactly what I do in the rest of this book. Again, not as a replacement for drugs, but as a way to drive our LDL as low as possible with our fridge and pantry in *addition* to anything we might have in our medicine cabinet.

Fiber and Phytosterols Flush Cholesterol

Dietary cholesterol is only found in animal-derived foods. Even if our diet were completely free of meat, eggs, and dairy, however, we can still absorb too much cholesterol from our digestive tract. Remember, the gut acts as a pressure release valve and serves as the dumping ground where our liver deposits excess cholesterol. Even if our cholesterol intake is zero, our liver releases surplus cholesterol into our intestine through the bile, expecting there to be around 100 grams of fiber to trap it and flush it from our body. Throughout evolution, we ate such an enormous quantity of plant foods that, based in part on studies of human coprolites,[123] that is, fossilized feces (paleopoo!), our ancient ancestors may have consumed grams of fiber in the triple digits each day.[124] That's more than five times that of the average American today.[125] So, when we get five times less fiber than nature intended, much of that excess cholesterol our body tries to get rid of gets reabsorbed and can circulate back through our system.[126] That's why one component of the Portfolio Diet is foods like oatmeal, high in the sticky fiber that helps trap cholesterol.[127] Where do the plant sterols fit in?

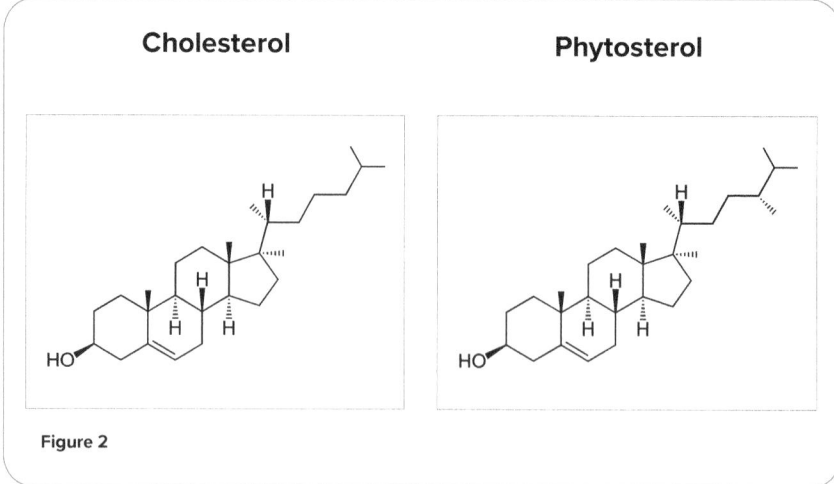

Figure 2

As you can see in Figure 2, cholesterol and plant sterols can look almost identical.[128] So alike, in fact, that the cholesterol receptors in the lining of our intestine cannot tell the difference. So, plant sterols compete with cholesterol to squeeze through the receptors. If there are a lot of plant sterols in our gut, some of the cholesterol can't get through and ends up in the toilet instead of in our bloodstream.

Figure 3 shows "fecal cholesterol excretion" in people eating different amounts of plant sterols on the same diet. In black is the amount of dietary cholesterol that's being pooped out, and in white is the amount of cholesterol dumped by the liver into the intestines that gets appropriately dumped in the toilet.[129] With increasing plant sterol consumption, increasing amounts of cholesterol are flushed out of the body. Note that even if you eat a strictly plant-based diet without any dietary cholesterol, you'd still be getting rid of more cholesterol by eating more plant sterols.

Where Are Plant Sterols Found?

Unfortunately, as with fiber, our intake of plant sterols has plummeted in modern diets.[130] We probably evolved getting about 1,000 milligrams a day, but, these days, we may be getting only about 300 milligrams, though those who eat more plant foods may get twice that each day.[131] Small amounts are found throughout the plant kingdom in vegetables, grains, legumes, and fruits,[132] but the highest whole-food sources tend to be nuts and seeds.[133] In

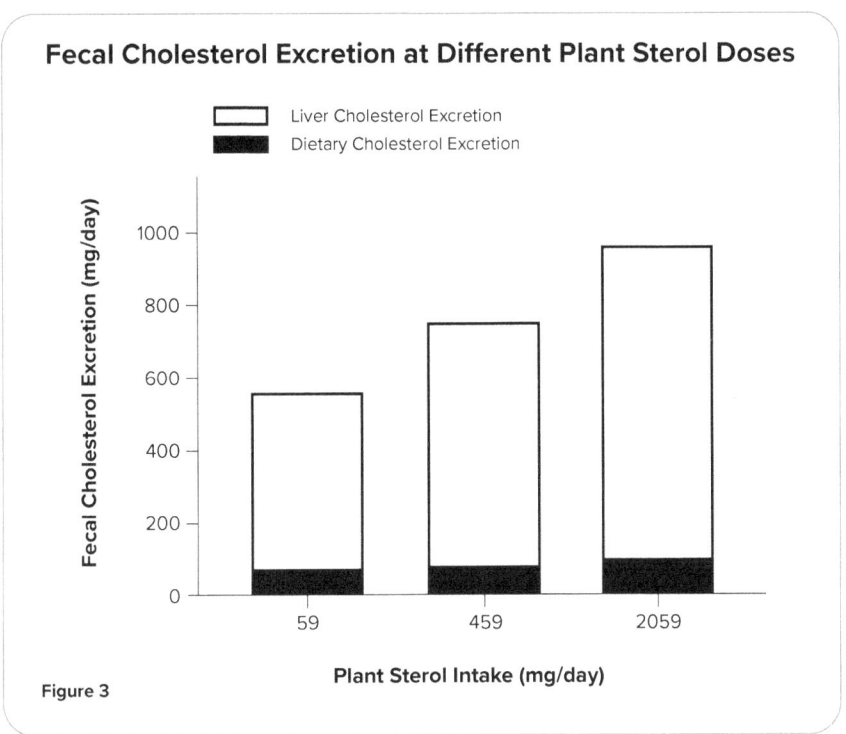

Figure 3

fact, plant sterols may help explain some of the cholesterol-lowering effects of nuts.[134] Nuts are already part of the Portfolio Diet. Why then add extra plant sterols?[135] Nuts may only get us a few hundred milligrams a day.[136]

As you can see in Figure 3, comparing the second bar to the first, eating lots of plant foods can draw more cholesterol out of our body than eating fewer plant foods, but getting 2 grams of plant sterols a day, represented by that third bar, can draw out even more.[137] And, as you can see in Figure 4, this translates into lower LDL cholesterol levels in our blood. So, the amount of plant sterols in a very healthy diet may drop our LDL by about 6%, but getting 2 or 3 daily grams of plant sterols can drop our LDL by around 10%.[138] That alone could reduce our risk of heart disease by about 10% over a decade or by 20% over a lifetime.[139] This is why multiple heart health clinical practice guidelines recommend the use of plant sterols to lower cholesterol, along with diet and lifestyle improvements.[140]

Plant sterols have been shown to be effective, but are they safe to take?[141]

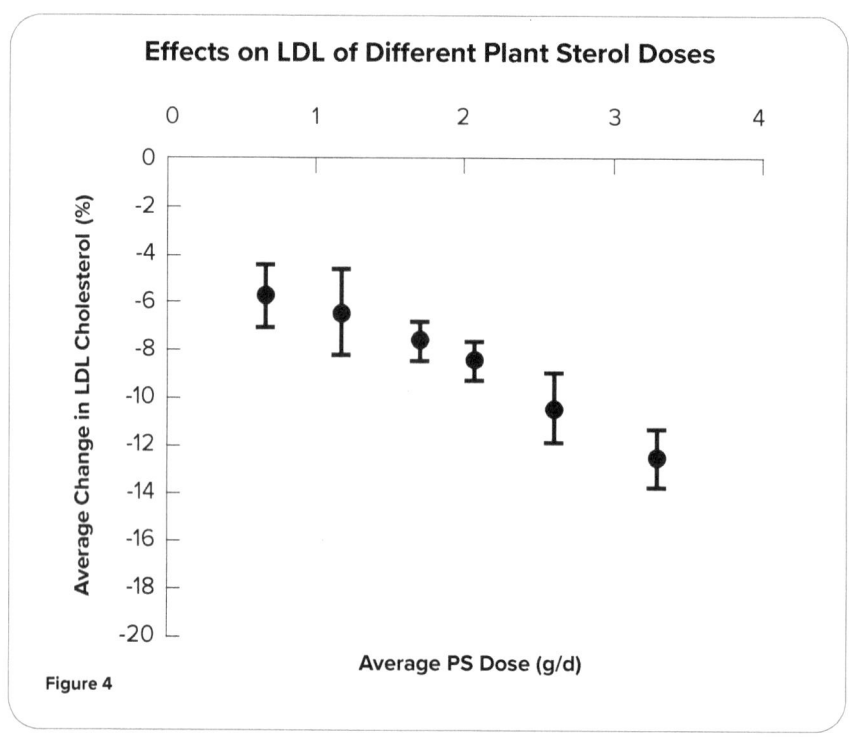

Figure 4

Plant Sterols Safety

Post-marketing surveillance studies are reported to have given plant sterols a clean bill of health,[142] based on feedback from thousands of consumers, but the studies were conducted by the company selling those products, so I don't take much comfort from them.[143]

Can Plant Sterols Also Take on Our Second Leading Killer?

According to an expert consensus statement from the European Atherosclerosis Society, at the recommended daily intake of 2 grams of plant sterols a day, "the available evidence does not suggest any adverse effect associated with long-term intake. Rather, evidence from animal and cell studies suggests a protective role of plant sterol intake and risk of certain cancers."[144] Population studies have also found a protective association between dietary phytosterol intake and lower cancer risk. Those who consumed the most had a 37% lower risk of cancer,[145] but where are phytosterols found? Healthy foods like nuts and seeds.[146]

Just a single ounce of nuts a day is associated with less cardiovascular disease and a lower risk of dying from cancer and all causes put together.[147] So, plant sterols may just be a marker for healthy food intake, though it's also possible that plant sterols may be one of the reasons nuts and seeds are so good for us.

There is a new class of anti-cancer agents known as *histone deacetylase inhibitors*,[148] which are available now for the low, low cost of $38,000 a month.[149] Plant sterols are the most potent *naturally* occurring such inhibitors reported to date, another reason offered for why plant foods may be so good for us.[150]

Interference with Fat-Soluble Vitamin Absorption

There is a worry that plant sterols could reduce the absorption of certain fat-soluble vitamins. They don't seem to impact concentrations of blood levels of vitamins A, D, or K, but they can reduce vitamin E levels by about 10%.[151] A greater concern has been about the loss of carotenoids, such as beta carotene. One modeling study suggests that if margarines become 100% fortified with plant sterols, the incidence in night-blindness—difficulty seeing in dim light—may increase by as much as 19 in 1,000 every year. At the same time, 1 in 1,000 would not get heart disease. Since night-blindness is considered a relatively minor visual disturbance, the benefits of fortification were said to "clearly outweigh any putative risks,"[152] but there is no need for any risk at all, because the relatively small suppression of plasma carotenoid levels can be countered by just eating more fruits and vegetables.[153]

Phytosterol Oxidation Products

The problem with fortifying a product like margarine with plant sterols is that it may be used in cooking, which could cause the plant sterols to oxidize into phytosterol oxidation products.[154] We know *cholesterol* oxidation products are particularly bad, but we aren't sure about oxidized phytosterols.[155] The bottom line is that we don't know enough about what happens when we heat them,[156] so it's better to be safe than sorry.[157] Don't cook with phytosterol-fortified products.

Red Blood Cell Fragility?

There was a concerning finding in rats, where plant sterols were found to make their red blood cells more fragile.[158] But, the opposite was found in mice; their red blood cells became *less* fragile.[159] And hamsters? There didn't seem to be any effect.[160] So, are we more like rats, mice, or hamsters? The amount of plant sterols researchers used with the rats was about 50 times higher than what we'd see with people. When put to the test with humans, it turns out there doesn't appear to be any issue with blood cell fragility.[161]

Cautionary Tale from Phytosterolemia?

There is a rare genetic condition called *phytosterolemia*, where people have extremely high levels of plant sterols in their blood and horrific heart disease, even as children.[162] This raised alarm bells that too many plant sterols, just like too many animal sterols (cholesterol), may be harmful.[163] But the same mutations that allow for the increased absorption of plant sterols also allow for the increased absorption of cholesterol, so these affected kids end up with cholesterol levels in the 700s mg/dL.[164] No wonder they're dying of heart attacks.

When those who genetically have higher levels of plant sterols in their bloodstream end up with higher rates of cardiovascular disease,[165] it's not necessarily because plant sterols are a problem.[166] Rather, those individuals are also absorbing extra cholesterol.[167] These genetic variations in sterol transporters, which result in increased blood levels of plant sterols and increased intestinal cholesterol absorption, subsequently result in higher LDL cholesterol levels.[168] In fact, that's how we estimate how efficient people are at absorbing cholesterol—by seeing how many plant sterols they have in their blood.[169] So, individuals with lots of plant sterols in their blood also have markedly elevated LDL cholesterol. No wonder they're at risk for heart disease.[170]

This increase in cholesterol absorption doesn't fully explain the increased risk, though, so it's possible that plant sterols may indeed contribute directly to heart disease. This has raised questions about the safety of supplementing food with plant sterols for the purpose of cardiovascular risk reduction.[171] However, the decrease in LDL achieved by the consumption of phytosterol-enriched foods is 20 to 40 times greater than the increase in plant sterols in the blood.[172] Thus, plant sterols would need to cause 20 to 40 times more atherosclerosis to cancel out their positive effect on cholesterol reduction, but there is no evidence for this. In fact, at the levels we get in our blood from consuming a few grams of plant sterols a day, there is no association with cardiovascular events in population studies.[173] This is why we get scientific consensus panel assurances that plant sterols are safe.[174]

Do Plant Sterols Actually Prevent Heart Attacks?

Although there is vast literature on plant sterols lowering blood cholesterol levels, to date, no study has investigated "the ultimate proof of efficacy: lowering the incidence of coronary heart disease."[175] There are no studies with hard clinical endpoints to confirm that the drop in LDL cholesterol from plant sterols translates to a drop in heart attacks. That is probably the strongest argument questioning recommendations for widespread use. The reason these studies haven't been conducted is that they are "hardly feasible." Even if participants had a baseline ten-year cardiovascular risk of 10%, more than 30,000 people would have to be randomized to plant sterols for a decade to detect such an effect.[176] At a more reasonable ten-year risk of 5%, more than 300,000 people might have to be enrolled.[177]

One could argue that plant sterols lowering cholesterol is all we need to know, since "clear evidence shows that lowering cholesterol concentrations by any mechanism is always accompanied by proportional reduction in cardiovascular risk."[178] This has been demonstrated with statins, other kinds of drugs, diet, cholesterol-lowering surgery,[179] and even through directly filtering LDL out of the blood.[180] One trial of extended-release niacin is cited as an exception, though. A group of patients with LDL levels starting down in the low 60s mg/dL achieved a further ten-point drop after a few years. That should have reduced their risk by at least 5% or 6%, but it only resulted in a 4% drop in events that didn't reach statistical significance.[181] So, even the one cited exception to the rule—anything that lowers LDL lowers cardiovascular events—lowered events (albeit not significantly).

Ezetimibe is a drug with a similar mechanism of action as plant sterols—that is, blocking cholesterol absorption.[182] It partially blocks the cholesterol absorption receptor, effectively reducing cholesterol absorption by about 50%. When it was put to the test, it did indeed significantly improve cardiovascular outcomes.[183] And the 13-point drop in LDL achieved by blocking cholesterol absorption with the drug is almost the same as the drop in LDL we'd expect from blocking cholesterol absorption with plant sterols, based on more than a hundred randomized controlled trials.[184] As such, we can be reasonably confident that plant sterols should indeed reduce our risk of getting cardiovascular disease.

This is the case even when we are already on cholesterol-lowering drugs or diets. What's more, blocking cholesterol absorption works even if we don't consume *any* cholesterol because the bulk of the cholesterol flowing through our digestive tract is not from what we eat, but from our own liver's production.[185] It also works for those on statin drugs.[186] In fact, adding 2 grams of plant sterols a day to what you normally eat may be equivalent to quadrupling your statin dose.[187]

The Best Dosing of Plant Sterols

The recommended daily dose of plant sterols is 2 to 3 grams a day,[188] based on dose-response curves showing that's where LDL-lowering benefit plateaus.[189] There's a comparable benefit curve with plant *stanols*, which are similar molecules.[190]

Plant sterols and stanols are absorbed better if taken with food[191] to coincide with the discharge of cholesterol-rich bile into the intestine with mealtime gallbladder contraction, along with any dietary cholesterol present. The same dose of plant sterols may more than double its LDL-lowering effect when taken with meals, rather than between them.[192]

The full LDL-cholesterol-lowering effect can be detected after just two weeks and presumably lasts as long as they're part of the diet. But, as soon as you stop consuming plant sterols and stanols, their cholesterol-lowering effect is lost within a week or two.[193]

The Best Source of Plant Sterols

Plant sterols in those kinds of doses are available in supplements and in fortified foods, which equivalently lower LDL by about 12 mg/dL.[194] The margarines are a non-starter. Are there any *healthy* phytosterol-fortified foods?[195] In Australia, there's a plant sterol-fortified shredded wheat called Weet-Bix, but I don't know if you can get it anywhere else.[196] Unless you live down under, the best option would seem to be plant sterol supplements.

It's always good to have third-party certification of authenticity for dietary supplements,[197] though I think there's only one USP-certified brand at the moment.[198] ConsumerLab.com tested and approved three others, though.[199,200,201] They're all fairly expensive (starting at 30 cents a day), so I was excited to learn plant sterols are available in bulk.[202,203] I presumed I could just sprinkle a bit on my food, but that presumption may be wrong.

As crystalline powder, it is much less efficient at inhibiting cholesterol,[204] which is why initial studies conducted half a century ago used high doses around 10 to 20 grams a day.[205] Researchers then figured out how to make these "free" sterols more soluble by creating sterol *esters*, which are what're now found in most supplements.[206] Some studies suggest that free sterols block cholesterol absorption as much as esterified sterols, but that was only after adding a large dose of an emulsifier to improve absorption.[207] A study showing that free sterols could lower LDL similarly relied on some proprietary means for solubilizing it.[208] So, I wouldn't recommend using the bulk powder form. (Just for fun, I tried taking the powder for a month and indeed saw zero effect, whereas I got a nice 17% drop in LDL from taking the exact same dose in encapsulated ester form.)

I'm not normally big on laboratory tests, but if you do start phytosterol supplements, I would suggest getting your cholesterol tested before and after taking them for about a month. LDL levels of some individuals respond immediately with a major drop, while others are more resistant or completely unaffected by plant sterol supplementation[209]—or even worse. The average response is around a 10% drop in LDL cholesterol, but you may get lucky and respond even better. Some get up to a 38% drop in their LDL. But it's also possible you won't respond at all, or your cholesterol might even go up. Some experience an *increase* in LDL by as much as 33%.[210] So, even though the average effect is favorable, you want to make sure it's working for you. You should be able to get your cholesterol screened for free through your doctor's office. These days, however, free or low-cost testing is available without insurance or a doctor visit. Check out, for example, www.attackheartdisease.com/free-ldl-c-test.

Cholesterol-Lowering Supplements to Avoid

According to cholesterol-lowering guidelines, dietary modifications are the cornerstone to controlling our LDL, but what about other dietary supplements?[211] For many of them, the evidence is sketchy.[212] A perfect example is policosanol.

No to Policosanol

Policosanol is a waxy extract from sugarcane found in a meta-analysis to lower LDL cholesterol by 24% over placebo.[213] Policosanol can even purportedly rival or beat a statin drug for lowering cholesterol.[214]

Given that policosanol works more than twice as well as phytosterol supplements at a fraction of the cost, why don't I recommend it?[215] More than 50 studies have reported substantial reductions in cholesterol with as little as 2 milligrams of policosanol; in comparison, it takes a thousand times that dose—2 grams of plant sterols—to have less than half the effect.[216] However, almost all of those studies were sponsored by the commercial enterprise in Cuba that markets policosanol.[217]

Independent researchers failed to replicate the results. They didn't use the exact same formulation, though.[218] Cuban researchers continued to claim that policosanol's efficacy is attributable to the unique purity and composition of their own preparation.[219] So, another study was set up to independently test the authentic Cuban policosanol preparation, and, low and behold, it did not work at all. The researchers used 10 milligrams, which is a typical dose.[220] Another independent study tried up to eight times that dose and saw a drop in LDL between 2% and 8%, but the placebo group also had an 8% drop, so all the policosanol doses flopped compared to a sugar pill.[221]

By 2009, the jig was up, exemplified by reviews with titles like "Policosanols lose their lustre as cholesterol-lowering agents."[222] But if someone didn't know any better and just checked the latest meta-analysis of randomized controlled trials, they'd see a significant drop in LDL cholesterol on par with statin drugs and might be duped into buying some. They would have to know to look at the subgroup analyses, which would inform them that the remarkable 55-point drop in LDL cholesterol deflates down to zero in the studies performed by researchers who hadn't been paid to promote policosanol supplements.[223]

When it comes to nutritional supplements and blood cholesterol, does anything work? Yes, red yeast rice and plant sterols.[224] I've discussed why plant sterols may be a good idea. What about red yeast rice?

No to Red Yeast Rice

Red yeast rice extract, produced by a purplish-red mold, is one of the only cholesterol-lowering dietary supplements shown to actually reduce the risk of cardiovascular events.[225] Based on studies including more than 10,000 heart disease patients, red yeast rice extract halved the risk of a subsequent heart attack and significantly decreased not just sudden death,[226] but premature death in general.[227] This isn't surprising, since it can decrease LDL cholesterol by an average of 36 points, which is comparable to what's seen with low doses of cholesterol-lowering statin drugs. That isn't surprising either, since it *is* a statin drug.[228] The mold produces lovastatin, the identical compound in the pill sold as Mevacor. In fact, that's how the drug was first produced, by having that very mold make it.[229] No wonder it's lowering cholesterol and saving lives.

So, are red yeast rice supplements suitable substitutes for statins? Unfortunately, no. There is such a large variability in statin content in red yeast rice supplements that predicting or understanding dose-related efficacy and safety is practically impossible.[230] For example, in one study, researchers investigated the variability in strength of 28 brands of red yeast rice supplements purchased from the mainstream retailers GNC, Walgreens, Walmart, and Whole Foods. No lovastatin was detected at all in 2 brands and its quantity ranged more than 60-fold in the other 26 brands.[231] Following the manufacturers' recommendations for daily servings, the quantity consumed per day would range more than a hundredfold. In the United States, supplement manufacturers don't list the amount of lovastatin,[232] but in Europe where they do, not a single supplement had values that matched what was on its label. Nine products had lower content, 24 had higher, and 3 had basically none at all.[233] So, as the researchers concluded, "Buyer Beware!"[234]

Ten popular red yeast rice products were recently analyzed by an independent U.S. laboratory, and most did not contain any lovastatin. And these results were worse than in previous rounds of testing in 2018 and 2010.[235]

Wide inscrutable variability isn't even the biggest issue with red yeast rice supplements. The recent analysis also found that approximately 30% were contaminated with a mold toxin called *citrinin* and one product exceeded the allowable safety limit by 65-fold.[236]

The U.S. Food and Drug Administration has been warning consumers for years to avoid red yeast rice products because of possible contamination with citrinin,[237] considered toxic to kidneys, liver, and fetus.[238] Citrinin has been found contaminating up to 80% of red yeast rice products.[239] Given that it's also classified as a genotoxic (DNA-damaging) compound, Europe restricted the maximum amount permitted in food supplements to 100 µg/kg.[240]

How many exceed that precautionary threshold? Thirty-seven brands of red yeast rice supplements were screened and 97% exceeded the safety limit—36 out of 37 supplements. Only one product was compliant. What's more, all of them contained the toxin, even though four of the contaminated products were explicitly labeled as "citrinin free." A risk assessment concluded that the toxin is "almost always present in red rice supplement samples, with values often higher than the legal limit."[241]

In Japan, there was a recent outbreak of serious kidney problems linked to red yeast rice supplements causing hundreds of hospitalizations and five deaths.[242] This rash of kidney damage was particularly alarming because the supplement manufacturer (Kobayashi Pharmaceutical) was using a strain reportedly incapable of producing citrinin.[243] An investigation concluded that the batch was contaminated by a blue mold that made a different kind of kidney toxin.[244]

As far as I'm concerned, if you choose to take a statin, take a regulated statin drug, not an unregulated statin supplement. Then, at least by law, you know how much you're getting and don't have to worry about mold toxin contamination issues. As a former chair of the Cleveland Clinic cardiology department concluded:

> *Modern medicine contains multiple examples...of 'natural' substances whose active ingredients were identified, isolated, studied, standardized, and regulated to create a product whose net benefits outweigh the harms. Without these steps, we are left relying on anecdotes, hearsay, and blind faith that a substance will have its desired effect.*[245]

Cholesterol-Lowering Supplements to Consider

In sum, of all the cholesterol-lowering supplements, the best available evidence for efficacy is for plant sterols, which I suggest trying, and red yeast rice, which I strongly suggest avoiding.[246]

Psyllium Husk

Also considered as having an "A" grade of evidence for efficacy is viscous soluble fiber, the sticky fiber featured in the Portfolio Diet, which recommends getting 20 grams a day from foods like barley, eggplant, oats, okra, apples, berries, or oranges.[247] Each serving of these foods has only a few grams, though, so getting 20 grams on a daily basis might be challenging.[248] That's where psyllium can help.

Powdered psyllium seed husk has more than 2 grams of viscous fiber per teaspoon.[249] Based on dozens of randomized controlled trials, psyllium, also known as *plantago* and sold commercially (with undesirable additives) as Metamucil, can reduce LDL cholesterol by 13 or 14 points. Psyllium *husk* works best, reducing LDL closer to 16 or 17 points.[250] In terms of dosage, one tablespoon a day should net you about a 10% drop in LDL.[251] Just make sure to follow the instructions and take it with lots of water.

Bergamot

DL, I've added two extra checkboxes for the two e- or 4-point drop in LDL could be considered "clinically important,"[252] a number of dietary supplements have been found to lower LDL cholesterol by more than 10 points:[253]

Effects on LDL Compared to Placebo

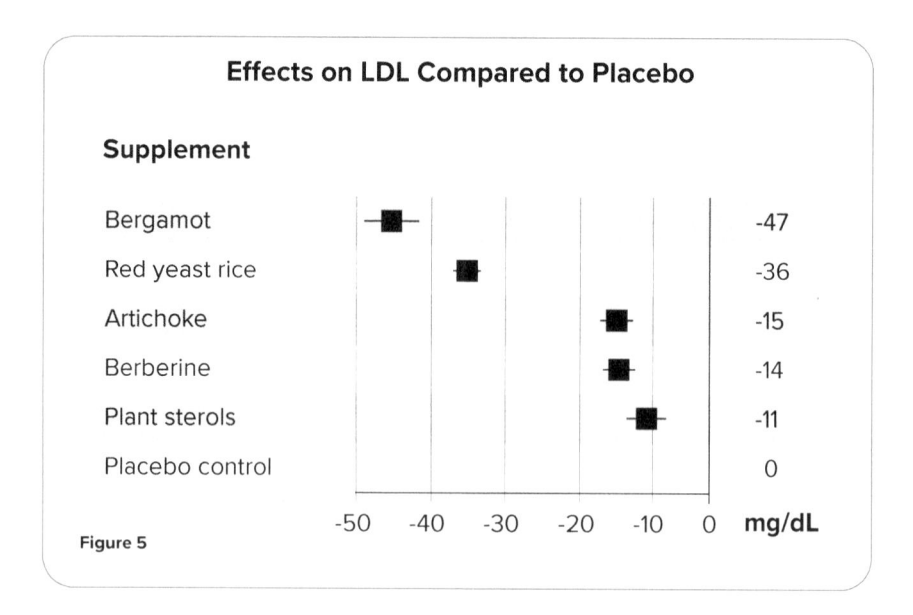

Supplement		mg/dL
Bergamot		-47
Red yeast rice		-36
Artichoke		-15
Berberine		-14
Plant sterols		-11
Placebo control		0

Figure 5

As you can see in Figure 5, bergamot appears to lead the pack,[254] though that's based on only half a dozen studies involving a few hundred people. Nevertheless, bergamot resulted in as much as a 55-point drop in LDL cholesterol,[255] likely because it seems to act like a PCSK9 inhibitor.[256] (See page 12.)

Are there any safety issues with bergamot? It contains *bergamottin*, which is one of the constituents of grapefruit that suppresses the detox enzymes in our liver and intestines, potentially increasing levels of certain drugs we may be taking. So, if you're on any medications, make sure to talk to your doctor before considering bergamot.[257]

There is a report of a case of intoxication with Earl Grey tea, which is black tea flavored with bergamot. A man had been drinking a gallon of Earl Grey a day and ended up with muscle cramps and twitches, thought to be due to a compound called *bergapten*, so don't drink a gallon of Earl Grey a day.[258] Larger doses of bergamot extract supplements don't necessarily have a larger effect, so if you do want to try it, I would recommend the lowest highly effective dose of 500 milligrams a day. The latest study used only 375 daily milligrams but only achieved half the effect.[259]

Artichoke

As you can see in Figure 5, artichoke leaf extracts are next on the list.[260] In 13 studies, researchers gave participants 50 to 2,700 milligrams of artichoke extracts for a few months and saw drops in LDL of 17 or 18 points. Again, more is not necessarily better, with doses of 500 milligrams and less a day appearing to work as well as doses over 500 milligrams.[261] Of course, this is assuming there is actually artichoke in your artichoke supplement.

One study found that only three out of seven dietary artichoke supplements contained the amount of a purported active ingredient as listed,[262] and another found all sorts of issues—not only lower concentrations than expected, but nondisclosed fillers and other plants entirely.[263] As I've discussed, this is one of the problems with dietary supplements. They are so poorly regulated that it's hard to know what's actually in them. At the very least, you should test your cholesterol before and after starting a purported cholesterol-lowering supplement to make sure you're getting at least some benefit. Ideally, though, you'd use the whole food.

In the case of artichokes, that would be getting perhaps 100 grams of artichoke hearts a day, which is about half a cup.[264] I think they're delicious, but I haven't been able to find any canned or jarred artichoke hearts without added salt. The solution? Frozen! Look for no-salt-added artichoke hearts in the frozen vegetables section of your favorite grocery store.

Barberries for Berberine

Just as we can eat artichoke hearts instead of taking an artichoke extract supplement to lower our cholesterol, we can eat the whole food source of berberine by eating barberries.[265] A systematic review and meta-analysis of 18 randomized controlled trials involving more than a thousand participants found that taking 900 to 1,500 milligrams of berberine a day can reduce LDL cholesterol by about 18 points within one to six months.[266]

Of those 18 trials, 15 were done in China,[267] where systematic issues of research quality have surfaced,[268] leading China's own Food and Drug Administration to question the integrity of Chinese clinical research.[269] Its investigation found 80% of China's clinical trial data to be fraudulent, containing "fabricated, flawed, or inadequate data."[270] Research integrity is expected to improve under new laws in which Chinese researchers found faking data can face execution.[271] Ironically, Chinese studies on berberine supplements may have a better chance of being valid since berberine is regulated there as an over-the-counter drug instead of a supplement, so it is required to at least contain what it claims.[272]

U.S. researchers tested 15 berberine supplements and found that most—9 out of 15—failed to come within 10% of the declared doses on their labels. The quality of the berberine product appeared unrelated to the cost, as the ones containing at least 90% of the labeled amount of berberine were not significantly more expensive than those that did not.[273]

That was in 2017. A follow-up study published in 2023 of 18 berberine supplements bought online similarly found that about half failed to contain the claimed amount.[274] NOW, a berberine supplement manufacturer, claims to have tested more than 30 competing berberine brands and asserts that more than half contained less than 40% of the labeled amount and about one in five didn't have any berberine at all.[275] I didn't recognize any of the brands they tested, though, so they may have gone out of their way to find fly-by-night companies.

Is berberine safe? It's a potent inhibitor of drug detox enzymes in our body, so it can affect medication blood levels. For example, in one case, berberine led to acute liver injury in a 68-year-old man when it pushed the blood levels of his blood thinner Xarelto to toxic levels.[276] Again, if you're taking any medications, always ask your doctor *before* starting any kind of supplements.

Gastrointestinal symptoms, including abdominal pain, constipation, diarrhea, and bloating, have been found to be common side effects of taking berberine.[277] I certainly experienced them when I tried it. Berberine-induced diarrhea is associated with a disturbance of the gut microbiome, at least in rats, though, ironically, berberine's also been used to treat certain forms of infectious diarrhea. It can kill off bacteria, such as cholera, but it may kill off some good bugs, too.[278]

The side effects may be dose-dependent, so if berberine does cause you problems, you can try reducing the dose.[279] For me, that didn't help. Even low doses upset my stomach. The solution to both the purity issues and the stomach issues may be to get berberine in its whole food form, barberries.[280] You can find dried barberries in Middle Eastern spice stores or online. About 5% to 8% of the berry is pure berberine.[281] There doesn't appear to be a significant difference in cholesterol-lowering efficacy between doses above and below 1,000 milligrams. So, to get the minimum effective 900-milligram dose, you'd just need to eat about two tablespoons of dried barberries a day.[282]

One study found significant reductions in LDL cholesterol using less than two daily tablespoons, but rather than the more common red ones, they used purplish-black barberries, which I haven't been able to find domestically.[283]

Supplements vs. Statins

In 2023, the SPORT study out of the Cleveland Clinic was published in the *Journal of the American College of Cardiology*. In this case, SPORT stands for *supplements, placebo, or rosuvastatin*. Participants were randomized to a starting dose of the cholesterol-lowering statin drug rosuvastatin (sold as Crestor), a placebo, or one of six common supplements—fish oil, cinnamon, garlic, turmeric, plant sterols, or red yeast rice.[284] The researchers wanted to know how they compared in terms of lowering LDL cholesterol within one month.

The drug reduced LDL by an average of 35% compared to the sugar placebo pill. And the dietary supplements? Not a single one was able to significantly beat the placebo. In fact, garlic seemed to make matters worse on average.[285] See Figure 6's cascade plot for a more detailed view:

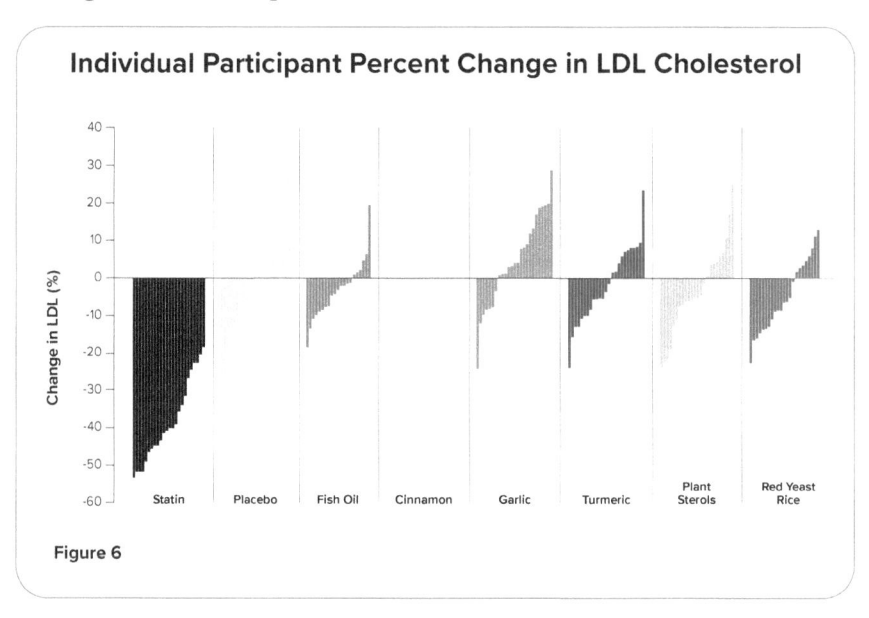

Figure 6: Individual Participant Percent Change in LDL Cholesterol

Each thin bar represents an individual participant. Start by looking at the placebo data. After one month of taking a sugar pill, LDL levels went up for about half the participants and down for the other half, just through normal month-to-month variation. The results for the six supplements look similar, suggesting they're not much better than the placebo sugar pill. With the garlic, note how more people ended up with higher LDL than lower, experiencing an average 5% rise. With the drug, though, the LDL cholesterol of every single participant taking the statin decreased by about 18% to more than 50%. Half dropped their LDL by 40% or more. "This clearly demonstrates," concluded the authors, "that every participant randomized to rosuvastatin had significant LDL-C[holesterol] lowering and all other studied products [the supplements] were almost akin to the flip of a coin whether LDL-C would increase or decrease."[286]

The study was not without its critics. First of all, what a peculiar mix of supplements to pick. Of the six dietary supplements examined, only three—plant sterols, red yeast rice, and garlic—are generally marketed as cholesterol-lowering.[287] The authors argue that fish oil and cinnamon make general heart health claims so a consumer might be duped into thinking they may lower cholesterol, but they don't have much to say about why they chose turmeric.[288] Why not bergamot, berberine, artichoke, or psyllium, which, as we know, have all been shown to be effective? Were the researchers just trying to make the drug look better by comparison? The trial was funded by the pharmaceutical company that sells Crestor,[289] but since it's been off-patent for about a decade, I assumed there wasn't much financial incentive—but I assumed wrong. Crestor still brings in more than a billion dollars a year,[290] which may explain why the researchers might have gone out of their way to pick some duds as comparators.

But shouldn't the red yeast rice have worked? Is it a coincidence that the brand[291] the researchers chose for its comparison study[292] was found to have zero active ingredients?[293] No wonder it failed. Their pick for plant sterols makes more sense, as it's one of the most common brands.[294] Why didn't it work? One commentator suggested the one-month timeframe of the study wasn't long enough,[295] but plant sterols should start having an effect within two weeks.[296] So, perhaps the particular brand they used (Cholest-Off Plus) just doesn't work very well.[297] It certainly has questionable ingredients like *carmine*, which is a red dye made out of crushed bugs.[298]

The timeframe issue may legitimately apply to the turmeric, though. Turmeric curcumin may decrease LDL a little, by about 6 points, but that's generally only been seen in studies lasting at least eight weeks.[299]

Why did the garlic *raise* LDL?[300] I thought garlic lowered it. In fact, less than an eighth of a teaspoon of garlic powder a day has been shown to be effective.[301] So why didn't garlic work in this study? Because it *wasn't* garlic; it was *Garlique*, a garlic extract supplement containing 15 other ingredients. It's also odor-free, so presumably some of the garlic compounds had been removed.[302]

The researchers did use real cinnamon,[303] but cinnamon,[304] like fish oil,[305] is not known to be cholesterol-lowering.

Despite the study's shortcomings, it did make an important point. Heart disease is life or death. We saw in Figure 6 what even a starting dose of a statin drug can do. In the face of overblown supplement claims and the mountain of misinformation surrounding statins, consumers may be hoodwinked away from taking "well-regulated, inexpensive, safe, and potentially life-saving medications with decades of supporting evidence."[306]

In sum, dietary supplements are so poorly regulated that we, as general consumers, can't ever be quite sure what's in them.[307] There's no guarantee that what's in a supplement actually matches what's on the label, which is why, whenever possible, whole foods are better. Artichoke hearts instead of artichoke extracts, barberries instead of berberine, and real garlic, like garlic powder, instead of garlic supplements. What other foods have cholesterol-lowering potential?

Foods That Lower Cholesterol

By sharply reducing our intake of the three main components that raise LDL cholesterol—saturated fat, trans fat, and dietary cholesterol[308]—most may be able to naturally achieve an LDL below 70 mg/dL,[309] which used to be the target for the primary prevention of heart disease.[310] For those who still didn't make the cut despite restricting their intake of meat, dairy, eggs, and processed foods, the next step was to add combinations of foods that actively pull cholesterol from our body, i.e., follow the Portfolio Diet.[311] But now that guidelines have shifted towards *the lower, the better* across the board, everyone should not only be lowering their intake of animal products and tropical oils, but also going out of their way to add cholesterol-lowering foods to their diet.[312]

See page 18 for the list of cholesterol-lowering foods featured in the Portfolio Diet.[313] How might we expand our portfolio? Let's start with tweaks

Dr. Greger's Daily Dozen

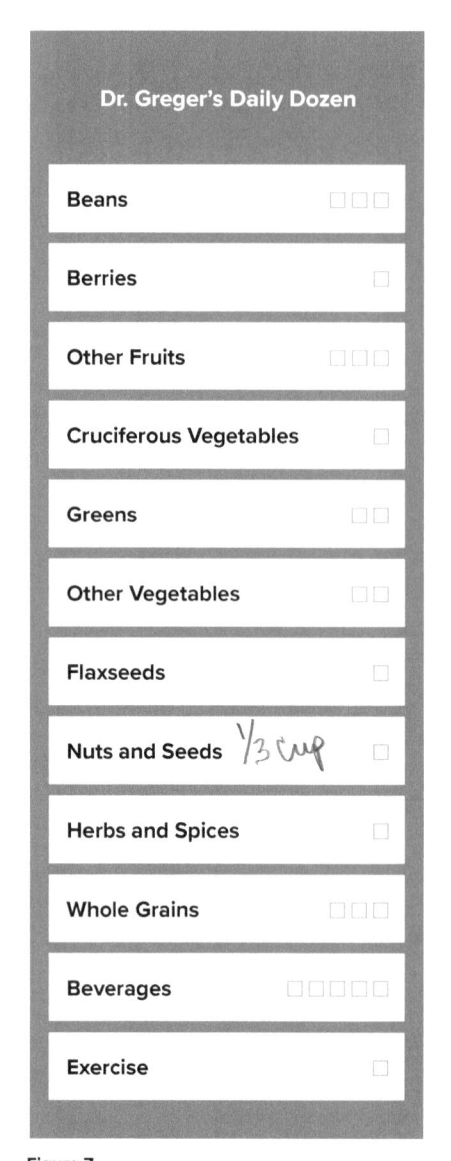

- Beans ☐☐☐
- Berries ☐
- Other Fruits ☐☐☐
- Cruciferous Vegetables ☐
- Greens ☐☐
- Other Vegetables ☐☐
- Flaxseeds ☐
- Nuts and Seeds ⅓ cup ☐
- Herbs and Spices ☐
- Whole Grains ☐☐☐
- Beverages ☐☐☐☐☐
- Exercise ☐

Figure 7

to the Daily Dozen,* the checklist that can help you incorporate some of the foods that I consider essential to an optimal diet:

Nuts

The handful of nuts I call for each day in the Daily Dozen doesn't quite cover the 45 daily grams recommended by the Portfolio Diet.[314] So, for optimal LDL-lowering, we may want to bump it up closer to a third of a cup a day. Are some nuts better than others?[315] Cashews and walnuts may be best for lowering LDL, with peanuts being least likely to be helpful.[316]

Of course, who can forget that wild study about brazil nuts I shared in *How Not to Die*? Researchers found that a single dose of 20 grams of brazil nuts dropped LDL cholesterol about 20% *within 24 hours*, and LDL stayed down for at least a month, suggesting that eating just four brazil nuts might be enough to improve LDL cholesterol levels for up to 30 days.[317] Not four brazil nuts once a day, but four brazil nuts once a *month*. In fact, eating four *every day* may put you at risk for selenium toxicity.[318] Even just one high-selenium brazil nut a day can increase the expression of pro-inflammatory genes.[319] Instead, if you have just the single

---

* I first presented this aspirational checklist in my book *How Not to Die* and it's since been developed into a free app for Android and Apple iOS. For details, you can get a copy of the book from your local public library or favorite bookseller and download the free "Dr. Greger's Daily Dozen" app.

serving of four brazil nuts once a *month*, you get a nice drop in inflammatory markers in your bloodstream within 24 hours with the benefits still evident a month later.[320] So, add a monthly dose of four brazil nuts to the list, along with getting your daily one-third cup of other nuts.

Beans

The Daily Dozen's recommended three servings of legumes a day help cover the plant protein requirement in the Portfolio Diet.[321] Is there a best bean? In the tenth anniversary edition of *How Not to Die*, coming out December 2025, I added black soybeans to my list of favorites, because the berry-like pigments found in the equivalent of just a tablespoon a day of cooked black soybeans can drop LDL cholesterol by 14 points over placebo within eight weeks.[322] So, let's add that to our daily diet as well.

You can buy black soybeans canned with no added salt or cook dried beans from scratch in about 45 minutes in an electric pressure cooker like an Instant Pot. One teaspoon of dried beans equals about one tablespoon cooked, so you could cook two-thirds of a cup of beans once a month and keep them in the freezer in silicone ice trays and pop out a "cube" every day to defrost for your daily tablespoon. Or, a single can will cover you for 28 days using the same drain-freeze-defrost method.[323]

Viscous Fiber and Plant Sterols

The other two components of the Portfolio Diet are 20 grams of viscous fiber and 2 grams of plant sterols.[324] Without even trying, the Daily Dozen should get you about 14 grams of viscous fiber a day. To make up for the gap, you can choose particularly rich sources from the various Daily Dozen categories. Consider prioritizing black beans, blackberries, apples, oranges, okra, eggplant, sweet potatoes, oats, and barley. You can also add to your daily diet a tablespoon of psyllium husk powder, which has 6 grams of viscous fiber. That alone should reach the 20 grams called for in the Portfolio Diet with even an unoptimized Daily Dozen. Just make sure you take the psyllium as directed with lots of water.

To complete the Portfolio Diet's portfolio, consider adding phytosterol supplements to your meals.[325] (See page 27.)

Barberries and Artichoke Hearts

In addition to the special nuts and beans, there are special berries. Two tablespoons a day of barberries should get you the 900 milligrams of berberine I mentioned earlier, though don't take them while pregnant or breastfeeding.[326] I encourage you to also consider including 100 grams of salt-free artichoke hearts a day as one of your two Other Vegetable servings in the Daily Dozen, which matches the cholesterol-lowering dose of artichoke leaf extracts.

Apples

Any other fruits proven in randomized controlled trials to lower LDL cholesterol? Dried figs flopped,[327] as did a mixture of dried fruits,[328] but half a dozen randomized controlled trials found that prunes, an average of seven a day, can drop LDL by 20 points.[329] Then, in 2024, The Prune Study was published, the largest prune study to date. After a year of participants eating up to 10 or 11 prunes a day, researchers found no benefit for cholesterol.[330]

Although there may be little cholesterol-lowering benefit from eating prunes, daily dried apples can drop LDL by as much as 24%.[331] So, consider adding two medium-sized apples or about a dozen dried apple rings to your daily diet as two of your three servings of Other Fruits in my Daily Dozen.

Flaxseeds

The Daily Dozen also recommends a tablespoon of ground flaxseed a day. Based on dozens of randomized controlled trials involving thousands of study participants, flaxseeds have been shown to lower LDL cholesterol,[332] but the smallest effective dose I could find in a controlled trial was 20 grams,[333] which is three tablespoons of ground flaxseeds. As you can see in the modified version of the Daily Dozen (Figure 8), tweaked to maximally lower LDL, I've added two extra checkboxes for the two extra tablespoons added for cholesterol-lowering purposes.

Dr. Greger's Maximally LDL-Lowering Daily Dozen

Beans ☐☐☐ including 1 Tbsp of black soybeans	**Nuts and Seeds** ☐ increased to a daily ⅓ cup, plus 4 brazil nuts *once a month*, not every day
Berries ☐ including 2 Tbsps dried barberries	
Other Fruits ☐☐☐ including 2 apples or 12 dried apple rings	**Spices** ☐☐☐☐☐☐☐ ¼ tsp turmeric ⅓ tsp amla ½ tsp sumac ¼ tsp black cumin 1/10 tsp garlic powder or ¼ clove of fresh garlic 1 tsp lemon balm powder ⅓ tsp ground savory
Cruciferous Vegetables ☐	
Greens ☐☐	
Other Vegetables ☐ including ½ cup of salt-free artichoke hearts	**Whole Grains** ☐☐☐
	Beverages ☐☐☐☐☐
Flaxseeds ☐☐☐ a total of 3 Tbsps	**Exercise** ☐

Figure 8

Herbs and Spices

For spices, my Daily Dozen calls for a quarter teaspoon of turmeric every day, along with any other herbs and spices you enjoy. How might we adjust this category to make it as cholesterol-lowering as possible?

Researchers found that amla, dried Indian gooseberry, may decrease LDL cholesterol by 25 points in 12 weeks. They used an amla extract, which might equal about a daily half teaspoon of amla powder.[334] When straight amla powder was tested, it appears a third of a daily teaspoon may decrease LDL by as much as 30 points or more.[335]

The spice sumac is another powdered berry. A gram or two a day of sumac can lower LDL by around 9 points.[336] The smallest effective dose would be about a daily half teaspoon, which is enough to significantly boost the efficacy of a statin drug by 11 points.[337] Note that sumac is in the cashew and mango family, so if you have an allergy to those, you may also be allergic to sumac.[338]

Dozens of randomized controlled trials involving thousands of participants found significant cholesterol benefits with nigella seeds, also known as black cumin. Researchers found that whole powdered seeds are more effective than extracted black seed oil,[339] and one study suggests that whole unground seeds are better than the powder.[340] The smallest effective dose is 500 milligrams, which is only about a daily quarter teaspoon of unground seeds or a pinch of ground black cumin, about a tenth of a teaspoon.[341]

Garlic powder can work at an even smaller dose, just 300 milligrams a day, which is about a tenth of a teaspoon of garlic powder or a quarter of a clove of fresh garlic.[342]

Fenugreek can also be considered a cholesterol-lowering medicinal plant, but the doses researchers used were huge.[343] The lowest effective dose I could find of the whole spice was 5 grams, four times a day, which is about five daily teaspoons of fenugreek powder—much more than culinary doses, which makes me concerned about long-term safety. The reason I even mention it is because the benefit was extraordinary, a drop in LDL cholesterol of more than 100 points compared to control.[344] I don't think I've ever seen a food do anything like that—reducing LDL by more than 50%. Hopefully we'll see future studies with more moderate doses.

The herb lemon balm can also help[345] at a dose of 3 grams a day, lowering LDL cholesterol by 13 points over placebo.[346] Drinking lemon balm *tea* does not appear to help, though,[347] and lemon balm may be unsafe during pregnancy.[348] Otherwise, we can add a daily teaspoon of lemon balm leaf powder to the list.

The herb savory, also known as summer savory, may be even more potent. A third of a teaspoon can reduce LDL by as much as 27 points over placebo,[349] so definitely consider adding that dose of ground savory to your daily diet as well. It's become quite the spice mix!

Figure 9 shows us where we are with the Daily Dozen after it's been optimized to lower cholesterol.

Feel free to pick and choose whichever spices you enjoy, but if the goal is to get our LDL as low as we can by using every possible safe and simple solution, how might we conveniently get as many of these as possible?

How Not to Die Recommendations (optimized to lower LDL)

Beans ☐☐☐
including 1 Tbsp of black soybeans

Berries ☐
including 2 Tbsps dried barberries

Other Fruits ☐☐☐
including 2 apples or 12 dried apple rings

Cruciferous Vegetables ☐

Greens ☐☐

Other Vegetables ☐
including ½ cup of salt-free artichoke hearts

Flaxseeds ☐☐☐
a total of 3 Tbsps

Nuts and Seeds ☐
increased to a daily ⅓ cup, plus 4 brazil nuts *once a month*, not every day

Spices ☐☐☐☐☐☐☐
¼ tsp turmeric
⅓ tsp amla
½ tsp sumac
¼ tsp black cumin
1/10 tsp garlic powder or ¼ clove of fresh garlic
1 tsp lemon balm powder
⅓ tsp ground savory

Whole Grains ☐☐☐

Beverages ☐☐☐☐☐

Exercise ☐

- **Vitamin B12-fortified foods or supplements**
- **± Vitamin D**
- **Seaweed**
- **± 250 mg algae DHA**
- **Psyllium husk powder** (1 Tbsp finely ground with sufficient water)
- **Plant sterols (2 g)**
- **± Bergamot extract (500 mg)**

How Not to Age Recommendations

- Vinegar
- Coffee
- Wheat germ
- Strawberries
- Pippali
- Green tea
- Potassium-based salt substitutes
- Chili peppers
- Mushrooms
- Purple sweet potatoes
- Pumpkin seeds
- Cranberries
- Nutritional yeast
- Cocoa powder
- Black sesame seeds
- ± Taurine

Figure 9

PUTTING IT ALL INTO PRACTICE

First, start by reducing or eliminating concentrated sources of the three components that primarily raise LDL cholesterol—saturated fat, trans fat, and dietary cholesterol. Cut down on meat, dairy, eggs, and processed foods containing partially hydrogenated or tropical oils, such as coconut oil, palm oil, and palm kernel oil.

That leaves us centering our diets around unprocessed plant foods. Some plants are even better than others, though, the inspiration for my Daily Dozen checklist.

As I detailed above, we can then tweak the Daily Dozen for maximal LDL-lowering by adding and prioritizing all the specific cholesterol busters. In sum, all beans and berries are good but adding that tablespoon of black soybeans and two tablespoons of dried barberries are particularly potent. All fruits and veggies are good, but we have the distinct data on the power of apples and artichokes for lowering LDL. Then we can incorporate brazil nuts (again, four a month, not four a day), bump up our daily intake of ground flax, and take those specific spices in those specific amounts.

In terms of supplements, in the appendix of *How Not to Die*, I emphasize the importance of a regular, reliable source of vitamin B12 and, if you don't get adequate sun, vitamin D, as well as a good source of iodine, such as seaweed. I also suggest considering taking a pollutant-free source of DHA. Adding to this list for cholesterol-lowering, consider supplementing with plant sterols (see page 27), psyllium, and bergamot extract (see page 31).

As if all of this isn't enough, my book *How Not to Age* introduced a list of potential anti-aging tweaks. For example, I recommended adding: vinegar to boost the enzyme AMPK; coffee to boost autophagy; wheat germ for the spermidine; strawberries and pippali, respectively, for the purported senolytic compounds fisetin and piperlongumine; green tea to boost Nrf2 defenses; potassium-based salt substitutes; mushrooms for ergothioneine; and chili peppers, purple sweet potatoes, pumpkin seeds, cranberries, nutritional yeast, cocoa powder, and black sesame seeds.* (Note that I'm skipping the cosmetic concoctions included in the book, like my recipes for topical vitamin C and nicotinamide facial serums, but adding the possibility of taurine supplementation, which was not included in *How Not to Age*. To decide if taurine is right for you, I did a webinar covering the risks and benefits that can be accessed at see.nf/taurine.)

Finally, if you are overweight, my book *How Not to Diet* features Twenty-One Tweaks to accelerate the loss of body fat.** For those who are above their ideal weight, every five pounds lost may lower LDL by about 2 points.[350]

Even without the weight-loss boosters, this is still a lot. How are we going to fit all of this into our daily routine?

Just as I developed the Daily Dozen to help me include the healthiest of healthy foods into my meals every day, I wanted to come up with a way to augment my Daily Dozen diet, incorporate anti-aging aspects, and take the Portfolio Diet to the next level.

Dr. Greger's Portfolio Plus Powder

My first step was to divide all the components into one of three categories: tasty, nasty, and neutral.

---

* Check out *How Not to Age* from your local library for details. If you want to buy a copy (in e-book, audiobook, or hardcover), note that 100% of the proceeds I receive from the sales of all my books (including this one!) are donated directly to charity.

** The free "Dr. Greger's Daily Dozen" app was modified to feature the Twenty-One Tweaks to accelerate weight-loss, based on the research from *How Not to Diet*. Users can toggle between the original Daily Dozen and the weight-loss focus.

Starting in Neutral Territory

It all began with ground flaxseed, a light nutty powder I could sprinkle on pretty much anything, so I always had a jar on my kitchen counter with a tablespoon scoop to remind me to check off my Daily Dozen box. When I learned about spermidine while researching for *How Not to Age*, I started mixing the flax with wheat germ and scooping twice to get a tablespoon of each. It's from that experience that I realized I don't mind sprinkling two tablespoons of a fairly neutral-tasting powder on a meal.

In that case, eating three times a day, I could accommodate six tablespoons of a bland powder every day. What in the lists on page 43 could I incorporate into such a mix to check off as many as possible at once? I imagined making a month's worth of such a powder at a time. Some people meal prep. I powder prep. Six tablespoons a day times 30 days equals 180 tablespoons of boosters I could incorporate into my diet as long as the taste is relatively benign.

The recommended three daily tablespoons of ground flaxseeds times 30 days equals 90 tablespoons, so half of the month's powder will be flax, 90 out of 180 tablespoons, about 5½ to 5¾ cups. I use preground brown flaxseed. Why brown? See my video *Golden vs. Brown Flaxseed Which Has More Benefits?* at see.nf/brownflax for details. Why preground? I used to buy bulk whole flaxseeds and grind a big batch in my blender until I learned that might contaminate the flax with billions of plastic particles.[351] A stainless-steel blender jar would take care of that, but it's spendy, around $100. Is it worth it? I don't know. There've been more than 15,000 papers published on microplastics since my last video series on the subject.[352] I have a lot of catching up to do, but that will have to wait for another book. In the meanwhile, I'll use preground flax.

So, the flax alone makes up 90 tablespoons of my monthly batch, but I still have room for another 90. Psyllium is also fairly neutral. The suggested daily tablespoon times 30 days equals 30 tablespoons of psyllium husk powder, about 1¾ to 2 cups. Single ingredient, finely ground, straight unflavored psyllium husks can be purchased in bulk online, which I consider much preferable to brand names like Metamucil that tend to contain fillers, sweeteners, colorings, and flavors. Note that since you'll be getting about a teaspoon of psyllium at each meal, make sure to also drink at least a cup of water each time.

There's still room for 60 more tablespoons of boosters. In *How Not to Age*, I noted that a single daily teaspoon of ground black sesame seeds can drop systolic blood pressures by 8 points over placebo, which, if sustained, could reduce the risk of a stroke by about 26%.[353] So, let's add that, too: a teaspoon a day times 30 days equals 30 teaspoons or 10 tablespoons, about ½ to ¾ cup. Ideally, we'd use raw black sesame seed powder. Most on the market is toasted, which may taste better, but it's healthier to eat raw nuts and seeds to reduce our exposure to advanced glycation end-products.*

Fifty tablespoons to go. What else can we add? I eat artichoke hearts in their whole-food form, but if you don't like the taste or can't find them salt-free, you could add five teaspoons of artichoke extract powder to get 500 milligrams a day. Unfortunately, there's no easy whole-food equivalent for the 500 milligrams of bergamot extract. (See page 31.) You could open up 15 grams of capsules and add them to the monthly powder batch, but I found that even with the ½ gram spread out across the six tablespoons of Portfolio Plus Powder taken each day, it was still too bitter. I mention it as an option only for those who don't like swallowing pills.

I like the sumac better. A daily half teaspoon works out to five tablespoons a month. If you aren't a fan of sumac's tartness, just add it to whatever you do with barberries, which have a similar sour fruity flavor.

If you decide to take taurine, four tablespoons of the pure powder added to the monthly batch will get you around 1,500 milligrams a day.

There are two sources of bulk phytosterol powder.[354,355] If you go that route, four tablespoons in the monthly batch would offer the recommended 2 grams a day. As I mentioned before, though, I'm skeptical that a powdered form will help (see page 27), so I take esterified plant sterol supplements three times a day to get my 2 grams.

What else? For iodine, I used to make veggie sushi a lot and, in the winter, love a bowl of miso soup with a little arame seaweed. I used to sprinkle about a half teaspoon of dulse on my meals, but even though dulse is pretty mild, I found it doesn't work with some dishes. Normally, I dissuade people from consuming kelp since we can risk iodine overload from more than a tiny amount, but a tiny amount would be perfect for our purposes here. There are brands that contain about 700 micrograms of iodine per gram

---

* See the Glycation chapter in *How Not to Age* for more detail.

of kelp powder, so two teaspoons spread out over the entire month will give us the recommended daily dose. Note that this is two teaspoons *a month*, which comes out to be about 1/16 of a teaspoon a day. It's so diluted in my monthly batch that I don't even taste it. If you already have a regular source of iodine, like if you use Eden brand* salt-free canned beans, there's no need to add this. I cook my beans from scratch in an Instant Pot and probably don't eat seaweed regularly enough, so I add it to my mix. Keep in mind that this strategy only works if the kelp powder is evenly distributed throughout the mix. This is even more important if you also want to try to get your vitamin B12 this way.

If you were to take vitamin B12 three times a day in the Portfolio Plus Powder, you would only need 2-microgram doses, whereas if you take B12 once a day, you need 50 micrograms. Once a week, you need a single 2,000-microgram dose.** By crushing up one 250-microgram tablet of cyanocobalamin, the preferred form of B12, and adding it to our monthly batch of powder, we'd theoretically get 2 to 3 micrograms per meal, but that's assuming it's perfectly evenly distributed. If you want to try taking your B12 in this mix, I'd suggest using at least a 500-microgram tablet. Is there any advantage to microdosing B12 throughout the day? One might argue it's more physiological to get tiny amounts over the course of a day, but I looked into the downsides of taking larger daily or weekly doses and didn't find any (see.nf/b12safety). So, the only real benefit of including B12 in this mix is not having to remember to take it in other forms.

Those are all the neutral components, so the final 44 or so tablespoons are dedicated to spermidine in the form of wheat germ, 2¾ cups, which offers close to 4 milligrams of spermidine a day. Here's the basic recipe, enough for an entire month:

Dr. Greger's Portfolio Plus Powder
90 Tbsps ground brown flaxseed meal
45 Tbsps wheat germ (raw)
30 Tbsps psyllium husk powder (finely ground)
10 Tbsps black sesame seed powder (raw)
5 Tbsps sumac

---

* Note that neither I nor NutritionFacts.org has ever accepted any money to promote any product from any for-profit company. Never have, never will.
** See our B12 infographic at see.nf/b12 for more details.

If you don't want to make a whole month's worth or want to make even more, just follow a ratio of 18:9:6:2:1 for those five ingredients in that order.

If you want to pack in even more, here's the extended recipe, again enough for an entire month:

Dr. Greger's Portfolio Plus+ Powder
90 Tbsps ground brown flaxseed meal
30 Tbsps psyllium husk powder (finely ground)
10 Tbsps black sesame seed powder (raw)
5 Tbsps sumac
± 4 Tbsps taurine
± 4 Tbsps plant sterols
± 5 tsps artichoke extract powder
± 15 grams bergamot extract
± 2 tsps kelp powder (assuming around 700 micrograms iodine per gram)
± 500 micrograms vitamin B12 (cyanocobalamin)
Wheat germ (raw) to fill the balance of the 180 Tbsps (11.25 cups) of the monthly batch

Store either recipe in an opaque, airtight container and make a habit of adding two tablespoons to every meal.

Next, Nasty

Now we turn to the louder powder. (*Disgust dust?*) Take amla, for example. It has a bitter, acrid, astringent taste. How are we going to get a third of a teaspoon of that a day? I used to disguise its flavor in smoothies until I discovered Japanese edible film, tissue-paper-thin, clear, tasteless squares, disks, or pouches made of pure potato starch. Edible film can be an easy way to swallow unappetizing powders without tasting them. Just put your third of a teaspoon of amla in the middle of the film, and, with dry hands, fold it like a wonton, dip it in water to seal it shut, then swallow with more water.

If you want to try this, I encourage you to start small and work your way up so you don't choke. I've grown comfortable taking a whole teaspoon's worth of powder at a time, so I use the opportunity to include the more strongly flavored components to create my BAT Powder, which stands for black cumin, amla, and turmeric:

BAT Powder
¼ teaspoon of black cumin
⅓ teaspoon of amla
¼ teaspoon of turmeric

Basically, you're taking approximately a teaspoon a day of a 3:4:3 ratio of black cumin, amla, and turmeric.

Edible film isn't your only option. You could also take unpleasant powders in prefilled capsules, fill capsules yourself with a capsule maker, or just make a shot—mix the powders with water and chug it down in what I call the "curry slurry method."

Lastly, Tasty

From the lists on page 43, the neutral components get sprinkled onto my meals in the Portfolio Plus Powder and the stronger flavors get tastelessly swallowed in my BAT Powder. The tastier items remain, which get folded into my regular meal rotation.

For example, during the winter months, I usually have a warm grain for breakfast like my Cran-Chocolate Pomegranate BROL Bowl (see.nf/bowl) or cooked oat groats with defrosted frozen mixed berries. Think of all the tasty things from lists on page 43 you can add. Lemon balm is in the mint family, so it pairs nicely. I like to mix it in a 1:3 ratio with freeze-dried strawberry powder and add a heaping tablespoon to whatever I'm having that morning. I make it chocolatey with cocoa powder, then add pumpkin seeds and nuts (and, on the first of every month, my four brazil nuts), two tablespoons of barberries, some chocolate balsamic vinegar, and, of course, two tablespoons of the Portfolio Plus Powder. Add a cup of coffee, and I can check off around 15 things from the lists.

For lunch, I've been into Italian-inspired cuisine recently, enjoying wholegrain pasta dishes like *hummac* (mac and cheese but with hummus instead of cheese). I can add the garlic, savory, artichokes, black soybeans, mushrooms, chili peppers, nutritional yeast, and potassium chloride as a salt substitute to tick off another ten items from the combined lists. Let's say you hate the taste of garlic and you like cooking Indian-inspired dishes. No problem. Replace the garlic with turmeric and make *BAG* powder instead of *BAT*. Make a lot of Middle Eastern? Add sumac to your food instead of the Portfolio Plus Powder.

In the afternoon, I have some green tea. Apples make a great dessert, and purple sweet potatoes can be a hearty snack or air-fried as fries as a side.

I take my BAT powder in the morning along with a capsule of plant sterol esters, bergamot extract, DHA, and vitamin D. Then I take an additional capsule of plant sterols at lunch and dinner, as well as the two tablespoons of B12-fortified Portfolio Plus Powder at each meal.

I don't have room in my edible film for the pippali and don't want to take two films a day. That will change, though, if the purported anti-aging benefit becomes more than theoretical. Likewise, if my ten-year risk of cardiovascular disease ever creeps up to 5%, I'd add a statin in a heartbeat. I'm still waiting on better human data for the taurine, but I think it's reasonable for those with a different risk tolerance to give it a try.

I can imagine how this could all seem a bit overwhelming, but you can benefit even if you take a few simple steps. Even if you just did one thing, like adding some apples to your diet.

Given the evidence that we should try to lower our LDL cholesterol as much as possible, I wanted to lay out every evidence-based tool I could find so you could mix and match them to have as much control over your destiny as you choose.

CONCLUSION

The number one killer of men and women? Heart disease. The primary driver of our number one killer? LDL cholesterol. No wonder nearly 100 million Americans are on cholesterol-lowering statin drugs.[356] When it comes to LDL, *the lower, the better*. So, in addition to whatever drugs you and your doctor may decide upon, ideally, we should all incorporate any and all safe, simple, side-effect-free steps that lower our LDL as far down as it will go. In this book, I've tried to identify every significant cholesterol-lowering food, herb, spice, and safe supplement to create a portfolio of things to do on a daily or monthly basis to drive our LDL cholesterol as low as possible.

The problem is it's quite a list—but that's a good thing. That means there is a lot we can do to lower our cholesterol, so pick and choose to figure out what works best for you. What I detailed above was my attempt to incorporate them all at the same time. That's how I've chosen to do it. This is not to say it's how *you* should do it. We each need to figure out what best fits into our life. I just wanted to share what I've come up with in case it gives you some ideas.

To track your progress, you can start by getting a free LDL cholesterol test by going to familyheart.org, thanks to the nonprofit Family Heart Foundation. It sends you the test in the mail. Then, you can have your doctor order tests every month to see how you're doing or find a testing center in your area like Quest or Labcorp and order your own. To save time, you could get an at-home cholesterol testing gizmo that uses drops of blood and gives you a digital readout in a few minutes. You can check it every week, try out different foods or supplements, and see what works best for you.

Whatever you do, however you test, let every heartbeat be a reminder to take better care of yourself.

From the bottom of my heart to your ever-healthier heart,

Michael

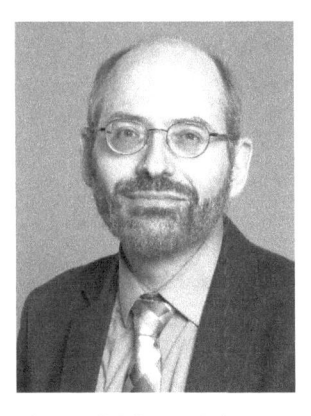

A founding member and fellow of the American College of Lifestyle Medicine, **MICHAEL GREGER**, M.D., FACLM is a physician, *New York Times* bestselling author, internationally recognized speaker on nutrition, and founder of the acclaimed nonprofit public health organization, NutritionFacts.org. He is a graduate of the Cornell University College of Agriculture and Life Sciences and Tufts University School of Medicine. All of the proceeds he receives from his books and speaking engagements are donated to charity.

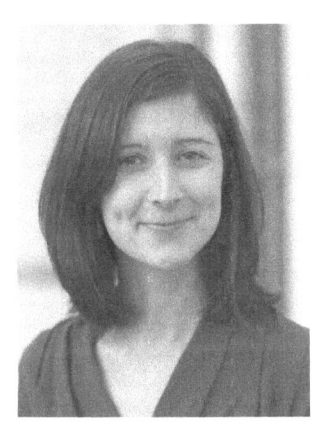

KRISTINE DENNIS, PhD, MPH, serves as the Senior Research Scientist of NutritionFacts.org. Prior to joining the organization, she spent more than a decade working in public health, designing and conducting research studies, and communicating scientific research. Dr. Dennis holds a PhD in nutrition and health sciences and a master's in public health from Emory University.

NutritionFacts.org

NOTES

1. Borén J, Chapman MJ, Krauss RM, et al. Low-density lipoproteins cause atherosclerotic cardiovascular disease: pathophysiological, genetic, and therapeutic insights: a consensus statement from the European Atherosclerosis Society Consensus Panel. *Eur Heart J*. 2020;41(24):2313–30. doi: 10.1093/eurheartj/ehz962

2. GBD 2021 US Burden of Disease Collaborators. The burden of diseases, injuries, and risk factors by state in the USA, 1990-2021: a systematic analysis for the Global Burden of Disease Study 2021 [published correction appears in *Lancet*. 2025 Jan 25;405(10475):302. doi: 10.1016/S0140-6736(25)00105-9]. *Lancet*. 2024;404(10469):231440. doi: 10.1016/S0140-6736(24)01446-6

3. Marston NA, Giugliano RP, Park JG, et al. Cardiovascular benefit of lowering low-density lipoprotein cholesterol below 40 mg/dL. *Circulation*. 2021;144(21):1732–4. doi: 10.1161/CIRCULATIONAHA.121.056536

4. Jones JE, Tang KS, Barseghian A, Wong ND. Evolution of more aggressive LDL-cholesterol targets and therapies for cardiovascular disease prevention. *J Clin Med*. 2023;12(23):7432. doi: 10.3390/jcm12237432

5. Laufs U, Dent R, Kostenuik PJ, Toth PP, Catapano AL, Chapman MJ. Why is hypercholesterolaemia so prevalent? A view from evolutionary medicine. *Eur Heart J*. 2019;40(33):2825–30. doi: 10.1093/eurheartj/ehy479

6. Atar D, Jukema JW, Molemans B, et al. New cardiovascular prevention guidelines: how to optimally manage dyslipidaemia and cardiovascular risk in 2021 in patients needing secondary prevention? *Atherosclerosis*. 2021;319:51–61. doi: 10.1016/j.atherosclerosis.2020.12.013

7. Mach F, Baigent C, Catapano AL, et al. 2019 ESC/EAS guidelines for the management of dyslipidaemias: lipid modification to reduce cardiovascular risk. *Eur Heart J*. 2020;41(1):111–88. doi: 10.1093/eurheartj/ehz455

8. Wang N, Fulcher J, Abeysuriya N, et al. Intensive LDL cholesterol-lowering treatment beyond current recommendations for the prevention of major vascular events: a systematic review and meta-analysis of randomised trials including 327,037 participants. *Lancet Diabetes Endocrinol*. 2020;8(1):36–49. doi: 10.1016/S2213-8587(19)30388-2

9   Fernández-Friera L, Fuster V, López-Melgar B, et al. Normal LDL-cholesterol levels are associated with subclinical atherosclerosis in the absence of risk factors. *J Am Coll Cardiol*. 2017;70(24):2979–91. doi: 10.1016/j.jacc.2017.10.024

10 Poli A, Catapano AL, Corsini A, et al. LDL-cholesterol control in the primary prevention of cardiovascular diseases: an expert opinion for clinicians and health professionals. *Nutr Metab Cardiovasc Dis*. 2023;33(2):245–57. doi: 10.1016/j.numecd.2022.10.001

11 Fernández-Friera L, Fuster V, López-Melgar B, et al. Normal LDL-cholesterol levels are associated with subclinical atherosclerosis in the absence of risk factors. *J Am Coll Cardiol*. 2017;70(24):2979–91. doi: 10.1016/j.jacc.2017.10.024

12 Hadjiphilippou S, Ray KK. Cholesterol-lowering agents. *Circ Res*. 2019;124(3):354–63. doi: 10.1161/CIRCRESAHA.118.313245

13 Heller DJ, Coxson PG, Penko J, et al. Evaluating the impact and cost-effectiveness of statin use guidelines for primary prevention of coronary heart disease and stroke. *Circulation*. 2017;136(12):1087–98. doi: 10.1161/CIRCULATIONAHA.117.027067

14 Byrne P, Cullinan J, Smith A, Smith SM. Statins for the primary prevention of cardiovascular disease: an overview of systematic reviews. *BMJ Open*. 2019;9(4):e023085. doi: 10.1136/bmjopen-2018-023085

15 Banach M, Reiner Ž, Surma S, et al. 2024 recommendations on the optimal use of lipid-lowering therapy in established atherosclerotic cardiovascular disease and following acute coronary syndromes: a position paper of the International Lipid Expert Panel (ILEP). *Drugs*. 2024;84(12):1541–77. doi: 10.1007/s40265-024-02105-5

16 Simonen P, Nylund L, Vartiainen E, et al. Heart-healthy diets including phytostanol ester consumption to reduce the risk of atherosclerotic cardiovascular diseases. A clinical review. *Lipids Health Dis*. 2024;23(1):341. doi: 10.1186/s12944-024-02330-7

17 Grundy SM, Stone NJ, Bailey AL, et al. 2018 AHA/ACC/AACVPR/AAPA/ABC/ACPM/ADA/AGS/APhA/ASPC/NLA/PCNA guideline on the management of blood cholesterol: a report of the American College of Cardiology/American Heart Association Task Force on Clinical Practice Guidelines. *Circulation*. 2019;139(25):e1082–143. doi: 10.1161/CIR.0000000000000625

18 Grundy SM, Stone NJ, Bailey AL, et al. 2018 AHA/ACC/AACVPR/AAPA/ABC/ACPM/ADA/AGS/APhA/ASPC/NLA/PCNA guideline on the management of blood cholesterol: a report of the American College of Cardiology/American Heart Association Task Force on Clinical Practice Guidelines. *Circulation*. 2019;139(25):e1082–143. doi: 10.1161/CIR.0000000000000625

19 Grundy SM, Stone NJ, Bailey AL, et al. 2018 AHA/ACC/AACVPR/AAPA/ABC/ACPM/ADA/AGS/APhA/ASPC/NLA/PCNA guideline on the management of blood cholesterol: a report of the American College of Cardiology/American Heart Association Task Force on Clinical Practice Guidelines. *Circulation*. 2019;139(25):e1082–143. doi: 10.1161/CIR.0000000000000625

20 Jaspers NEM, Ridker PM, Dorresteijn JAN, Visseren FLJ. The prediction of therapy-benefit for individual cardiovascular disease prevention: rationale, implications, and implementation. *Curr Opin Lipidol*. 2018;29(6):436–44. doi: 10.1097/MOL.0000000000000554

21 U-Prevent calculator. ORTEC. Updated April 8, 2025. Accessed April 28, 2025. https://u-prevent.com/

22   Barrett B, Ricco J, Wallace M, Kiefer D, Rakel D. Communicating statin evidence to support shared decision-making. *BMC Fam Pract*. 2016;17:41. doi: 10.1186/s12875-016-0436-9

23   Demasi M. Statin wars: have we been misled about the evidence? A narrative review. *Br J Sports Med*. 2018;52(14):905–9.

24   Trewby PN, Reddy AV, Trewby CS, Ashton VJ, Brennan G, Inglis J. Are preventive drugs preventive enough? A study of patients' expectation of benefit from preventive drugs. *Clin Med*. 2002;2(6):527–33. doi: 10.7861/clinmedicine.2-6-527

25   Diprose W, Verster F. The preventive-pill paradox: how shared decision making could increase cardiovascular morbidity and mortality. *Circulation*. 2016;134(21):1599–600. doi: 10.1161/CIRCULATIONAHA.116.025204

26   Trewby PN, Reddy AV, Trewby CS, Ashton VJ, Brennan G, Inglis J. Are preventive drugs preventive enough? A study of patients' expectation of benefit from preventive drugs. *Clin Med*. 2002;2(6):527–33. doi: 10.7861/clinmedicine.2-6-527

27   Pippin JJ. Primary prevention cardiovascular disease: better than drugs. *Arch Intern Med*. 2010;170(20):1860–1. doi: 10.1001/archinternmed.2010.402

28   Menkes DB, Mintzes B, Lexchin J. Direct-to-consumer advertising: a modifiable driver of overdiagnosis and overtreatment. *BMJ Evid Based Med*. 2024;29(6):423–5. doi: 10.1136/bmjebm-2023-112622

29   Borovcnik M. Risk and decision making: modeling and statistics in medicine – case studies. In: Sriraman B, ed. *Handbook of the Mathematics of the Arts and Sciences*. Springer International Publishing; 2019:1–36. doi: 10.1007/978-3-319-70658-0_126-1

30   Raittio E, Ashraf J, Farmer J, Nascimento GG, Aldossri M. Reporting of absolute and relative risk measures in oral health and cardiovascular events studies: a systematic review. *Community Dent Oral Epidemiol*. 2023;51(2):283–91. doi: 10.1111/cdoe.12738

31   Sever PS, Dahlöf B, Poulter NR, et al. Prevention of coronary and stroke events with atorvastatin in hypertensive patients who have average or lower-than-average cholesterol concentrations, in the Anglo-Scandinavian Cardiac Outcomes Trial—Lipid Lowering Arm (ASCOT-LLA): a multicentre randomised controlled trial. *Lancet*. 2003;361(9364):1149–58. doi: 10.1016/S0140-6736(03)12948-0

32   Byrne P, Demasi M, Jones M, Smith SM, O'Brien KK, DuBroff R. Evaluating the association between low-density lipoprotein cholesterol reduction and relative and absolute effects of statin treatment: a systematic review and meta-analysis. *JAMA Intern Med*. 2022;182(5):474–81. doi: 10.1001/jamainternmed.2022.0134

33   Albarqouni L, Doust J, Glasziou P. Patient preferences for cardiovascular preventive medication: a systematic review. *Heart*. 2017;103(20):1578–86. doi: 10.1136/heartjnl-2017-311244

34   Albarqouni L, Doust J, Glasziou P. Patient preferences for cardiovascular preventive medication: a systematic review. *Heart*. 2017;103(20):1578–86. doi: 10.1136/heartjnl-2017-311244

35   Fontana M, Asaria P, Moraldo M, et al. Patient-accessible tool for shared decision making in cardiovascular primary prevention: balancing longevity benefits against medication disutility. *Circulation*. 2014;129(24):2539–46. doi: 10.1161/CIRCULATIONAHA.113.007595

36 Halvorsen PA, Aasland OG, Kristiansen IS. Decisions on statin therapy by patients' opinions about survival gains: cross sectional survey of general practitioners. *BMC Fam Pract*. 2015;16:79. doi: 10.1186/s12875-015-0288-8

37 Durai V, Redberg RF. Statin therapy for the primary prevention of cardiovascular disease: cons. *Atherosclerosis*. 2022;356:46–9. doi: 10.1016/j.atherosclerosis.2022.07.003

38 Yourman LC, Cenzer IS, Boscardin WJ, et al. Evaluation of time to benefit of statins for the primary prevention of cardiovascular events in adults aged 50 to 75 years: a meta-analysis. *JAMA Intern Med*. 2021;181(2):179–85. doi: 10.1001/jamainternmed.2020.6084

39 Kostapanos MS, Elisaf MS. Statins and mortality: the untold story. *Br J Clin Pharmacol*. 2017;83(5):938–41. doi: 10.1111/bcp.13202

40 Durai V, Redberg RF. Statin therapy for the primary prevention of cardiovascular disease: cons. *Atherosclerosis*. 2022;356:46–9. doi: 10.1016/j.atherosclerosis.2022.07.003

41 Cai T, Abel L, Langford O, et al. Associations between statins and adverse events in primary prevention of cardiovascular disease: systematic review with pairwise, network, and dose-response meta-analyses. *BMJ*. 2021;374:n1537. doi: 10.1136/bmj.n1537

42 Preiss D, Seshasai SR, Welsh P, et al. Risk of incident diabetes with intensive-dose compared with moderate-dose statin therapy: a meta-analysis. *JAMA*. 2011;305(24):2556–64. doi: 10.1001/jama.2011.860

43 Ma W, Pan Q, Pan D, Xu T, Zhu H, Li D. Efficacy and safety of lipid-lowering drugs of different intensity on clinical outcomes: a systematic review and network meta-analysis. *Front Pharmacol*. 2021;12:713007. doi: 10.3389/fphar.2021.713007

44 Cai T, Abel L, Langford O, et al. Associations between statins and adverse events in primary prevention of cardiovascular disease: systematic review with pairwise, network, and dose-response meta-analyses. *BMJ*. 2021;374:n1537. doi: 10.1136/bmj.n1537

45 Masson W, Lobo M, Barbagelata L, Nogueira JP. Statins and new-onset diabetes in primary prevention setting: an updated meta-analysis stratified by baseline diabetes risk. *Acta Diabetol*. 2024;61(3):351–60. doi: 10.1007/s00592-023-02205-w

46 Kostapanos MS, Elisaf MS. Statins and mortality: the untold story. *Br J Clin Pharmacol*. 2017;83(5):938–41. doi: 10.1111/bcp.13202

47 Rikhi R, Shapiro MD. Impact of statin therapy on diabetes incidence: implications for primary prevention. *Curr Cardiol Rep*. 2024;26(12):1447–52. doi: 10.1007/s11886-024-02141-3

48 Bradley CK, Wang TY, Li S, et al. Patient-reported reasons for declining or discontinuing statin therapy: insights from the PALM registry. *J Am Heart Assoc*. 2019;8(7):e011765. doi: 10.1161/JAHA.118.011765

49 Hadjiphilippou S, Ray KK. Cholesterol-lowering agents. *Circ Res*. 2019;124(3):354–63. doi: 10.1161/CIRCRESAHA.118.313245

50 Yourman LC, Cenzer IS, Boscardin WJ, et al. Evaluation of time to benefit of statins for the primary prevention of cardiovascular events in adults aged 50 to 75 years: a meta-analysis. *JAMA Intern Med*. 2021;181(2):179–85. doi: 10.1001/jamainternmed.2020.6084

51. Volpe M, Patrono C. The cardiovascular benefits of statins outweigh adverse effects in primary prevention: results of a large systematic review and meta-analysis. *Eur Heart J.* 2021;42(44):4518–19. doi: 10.1093/eurheartj/ehab647

52. Volpe M, Patrono C. The cardiovascular benefits of statins outweigh adverse effects in primary prevention: results of a large systematic review and meta-analysis. *Eur Heart J.* 2021;42(44):4518–19. doi: 10.1093/eurheartj/ehab647

53. Barrett B, Ricco J, Wallace M, Kiefer D, Rakel D. Communicating statin evidence to support shared decision-making. *BMC Fam Pract.* 2016;17:41. doi: 10.1186/s12875-016-0436-9

54. Durai V, Redberg RF. Statin therapy for the primary prevention of cardiovascular disease: cons. *Atherosclerosis.* 2022;356:46–9. doi: 10.1016/j.atherosclerosis.2022.07.003

55. Malhotra A, Apps A, Capewell S. Maximising the benefits and minimising the harms of statins. *Prescriber.* 2015;26(1-2):6–7. doi: 10.1002/psb.1293

56. Durai V, Redberg RF. Statin therapy for the primary prevention of cardiovascular disease: cons. *Atherosclerosis.* 2022;356:46–9. doi: 10.1016/j.atherosclerosis.2022.07.003

57. Durai V, Redberg RF. Statin therapy for the primary prevention of cardiovascular disease: cons. *Atherosclerosis.* 2022;356:46–9. doi: 10.1016/j.atherosclerosis.2022.07.003

58. Ganga HV, Slim HB, Thompson PD. A systematic review of statin-induced muscle problems in clinical trials. *Am Heart J.* 2014;168(1):6–15. doi:10.1016/j.ahj.2014.03.019

59. Malhotra A, Apps A, Capewell S. Maximising the benefits and minimising the harms of statins. *Prescriber.* 2015;26(1-2):6–7. doi: 10.1002/psb.1293

60. Durai V, Redberg RF. Statin therapy for the primary prevention of cardiovascular disease: cons. *Atherosclerosis.* 2022;356:46–9. doi: 10.1016/j.atherosclerosis.2022.07.003

61. Durai V, Redberg RF. Statin therapy for the primary prevention of cardiovascular disease: cons. *Atherosclerosis.* 2022;356:46–9. doi: 10.1016/j.atherosclerosis.2022.07.003

62. Stroes ES, Thompson PD, Corsini A, et al. Statin-associated muscle symptoms: impact on statin therapy–European Atherosclerosis Society Consensus Panel Statement on Assessment, Aetiology and Management. *Eur Heart J.* 2015;36(17):1012–22. doi:10.1093/eurheartj/ehv043

63. Golomb BA. Misinterpretation of trial evidence on statin adverse effects may harm patients. *Eur J Prev Cardiol.* 2015;22(4):492–3. doi: 10.1177/2047487314533085

64. Golomb BA, Evans MA, Dimsdale JE, White HL. Effects of statins on energy and fatigue with exertion: results from a randomized controlled trial. *Arch Intern Med.* 2012;172(15):1180–2. doi: 10.1001/archinternmed.2012.2171

65. Farahani P. Sex/gender disparities in randomized controlled trials of statins: the impact of awareness efforts. *Clin Invest Med.* 2014;37(3):E163. doi: 10.25011/cim.v37i3.21383

66. Ornish D, Madison C, Kivipelto M, et al. Effects of intensive lifestyle changes on the progression of mild cognitive impairment or early dementia due to Alzheimer's disease: a randomized, controlled clinical trial. *Alzheimers Res Ther*. 2024;16(1):122. doi: 10.1186/s13195-024-01482-z

67. de Lorgeril M, Renaud S, Mamelle N, et al. Mediterranean alpha-linolenic acid-rich diet in secondary prevention of coronary heart disease. *Lancet*. 1994;343(8911):1454–9. doi: 10.1016/s0140-6736(94)92580-1

68. Ausiello D. Alexander Leaf. *Harvard Medical School: Memorial Minutes*. December 2012. Accessed July 6, 2025. https://fa.hms.harvard.edu/file_url/399

69. Leaf A. Dietary prevention of coronary heart disease: the Lyon Diet Heart Study. *Circulation*. 1999;99(6):733–5. doi: 10.1161/01.cir.99.6.733

70. Leaf A. Dietary prevention of coronary heart disease: the Lyon Diet Heart Study. *Circulation*. 1999;99(6):733–5. doi: 10.1161/01.cir.99.6.733

71. FDA drug safety communication: important safety label changes to cholesterol-lowering statin drugs. US Food and Drug Administration. February 28, 2012. Accessed July 6, 2025. https://www.fda.gov/drugs/drug-safety-and-availability/fda-drug-safety-communication-important-safety-label-changes-cholesterol-lowering-statin-drugs

72. Muldoon MF, Ryan CM, Sereika SM, Flory JD, Manuck SB. Randomized trial of the effects of simvastatin on cognitive functioning in hypercholesterolemic adults. *Am J Med*. 2004;117(11):823–9. doi: 10.1016/j.amjmed.2004.07.041

73. Muldoon MF, Barger SD, Ryan CM, et al. Effects of lovastatin on cognitive function and psychological well-being. *Am J Med*. 2000;108(7):538–46. doi: 10.1016/s0002-9343(00)00353-3

74. Kazibwe R, Rikhi R, Mirzai S, Ashburn NP, Schaich CL, Shapiro M. Do statins affect cognitive health? A narrative review and critical analysis of the evidence. *Curr Atheroscler Rep*. 2024;27(1):2. doi: 10.1007/s11883-024-01255-x

75. Ott BR, Daiello LA, Dahabreh IJ, et al. Do statins impair cognition? A systematic review and meta-analysis of randomized controlled trials. *J Gen Intern Med*. 2015;30(3):348–58. doi: 10.1007/s11606-014-3115-3

76. Westphal Filho FL, Moss Lopes PR, Menegaz de Almeida A, et al. Statin use and dementia risk: a systematic review and updated meta-analysis. *Alzheimers Dement*. 2025;11(1):e70039. doi: 10.1002/trc2.70039

77. Corsinovi L, Biasi F, Poli G, Leonarduzzi G, Isaia G. Dietary lipids and their oxidized products in Alzheimer's disease. *Mol Nutr Food Res*. 2011;55 Suppl 2:S161–72.

78. Lanfranco MF, Ng CA, Rebeck GW. ApoE lipidation as a therapeutic target in Alzheimer's disease. *Int J Mol Sci*. 2020;21(17):6336. doi:10.3390/ijms21176336

79. Westphal Filho FL, Moss Lopes PR, Menegaz de Almeida A, et al. Statin use and dementia risk: a systematic review and updated meta-analysis. *Alzheimers Dement*. 2025;11(1):e70039. doi: 10.1002/trc2.70039

80. Paparodis RD, Bantouna D, Livadas S, Angelopoulos N. Statin therapy in primary and secondary cardiovascular disease prevention. *Curr Atheroscler Rep*. 2024;27(1):21. doi: 10.1007/s11883-024-01265-9

81 Banach M, Surma S, Toth PP. 2023: the year in cardiovascular disease — the year of new and prospective lipid lowering therapies. Can we render dyslipidemia a rare disease by 2024? *Arch Med Sci*. 2023;19(6):1602–15. doi: 10.5114/aoms/174743

82 Mustad VA, Etherton TD, Cooper AD, et al. Reducing saturated fat intake is associated with increased levels of LDL receptors on mononuclear cells in healthy men and women. *J Lipid Res*. 1997;38(3):459–68. doi: 10.1016/S0022-2275(20)37254-0

83 Cohen JC, Boerwinkle E, Mosley TH, Hobbs HH. Sequence variations in PCSK9, low LDL, and protection against coronary heart disease. *N Engl J Med*. 2006;354(12):1264–72. doi: 10.1056/NEJMoa054013

84 Mustad VA, Etherton TD, Cooper AD, et al. Reducing saturated fat intake is associated with increased levels of LDL receptors on mononuclear cells in healthy men and women. *J Lipid Res*. 1997;38(3):459–68. doi: 10.1016/S0022-2275(20)37254-0

85 Smith KW, White CM. Inclisiran: a novel small interfering RNA drug for low-density lipoprotein reduction. *J Clin Pharmacol*. 2022;62(9):1079–85. doi:10.1002/jcph.2045

86 Awad K, Mikhailidis DP, Toth PP, et al. Efficacy and safety of alternate-day versus daily dosing of statins: a systematic review and meta-analysis. *Cardiovasc Drugs Ther*. 2017;31(4):419–31. doi: 10.1007/s10557-017-6743-0

87 Goldstein JL, Brown MS. Akira Endo, who discovered a "penicillin" for heart attacks (1933 to 2024). *Proc Natl Acad Sci USA*. 2024;121(40):e2416550121. doi: 10.1073/pnas.2416550121

88 Endo A. The discovery and development of HMG-CoA reductase inhibitors. *J Lipid Res*. 1992;33(11):1569–82. PMID: 1464741

89 Endo A. A gift from nature: the birth of the statins. *Nat Med*. 2008;14(10):1050–2. doi: 10.1038/nm1008-1050

90 Paparodis RD, Bantouna D, Livadas S, Angelopoulos N. Statin therapy in primary and secondary cardiovascular disease prevention. *Curr Atheroscler Rep*. 2024;27(1):21. doi: 10.1007/s11883-024-01265-9

91 Yebyo HG, Aschmann HE, Kaufmann M, Puhan MA. Comparative effectiveness and safety of statins as a class and of specific statins for primary prevention of cardiovascular disease: a systematic review, meta-analysis, and network meta-analysis of randomized trials with 94,283 participants. *Am Heart J*. 2019;210:18–28. doi: 10.1016/j.ahj.2018.12.007

92 Lessons from Lipitor and the broken blockbuster drug model. *Lancet*. 2011;378(9808):1976. doi: 10.1016/S0140-6736(11)61858-8

93 Arnett DK, Blumenthal RS, Albert MA, et al. 2019 ACC/AHA guideline on the primary prevention of cardiovascular disease: a report of the American College of Cardiology/American Heart Association Task Force on Clinical Practice Guidelines. *Circulation*. 2019;140(11):e596–646. doi: 10.1161/CIR.0000000000000678

94 Thompson PD, Panza G, Zaleski A, Taylor B. Statin-associated side effects. *J Am Coll Cardiol*. 2016;67(20):2395–410. doi: 10.1016/j.jacc.2016.02.071

95 Arnett DK, Blumenthal RS, Albert MA, et al. 2019 ACC/AHA guideline on the primary prevention of cardiovascular disease: a report of the American College of Cardiology/American Heart Association Task Force on Clinical Practice Guidelines. *Circulation*. 2019;140(11):e596–646. doi: 10.1161/CIR.0000000000000678

96   Kendall CW, Jenkins DJ. A dietary portfolio: maximal reduction of low-density lipoprotein cholesterol with diet. *Curr Atheroscler Rep*. 2004;6(6):492–8. doi: 10.1007/s11883-004-0091-9

97   Grundy SM. Does dietary cholesterol matter? *Curr Atheroscler Rep*. 2016;18(11):68. doi: 10.1007/s11883-016-0615-0

98   Trumbo PR, Shimakawa T. Tolerable upper intake levels for trans fat, saturated fat, and cholesterol. *Nutr Rev*. 2011;69(5):270–8. doi: 10.1111/j.1753-4887.2011.00389.x

99   National Cancer Institute. *Identification of Top Food Sources of Various Dietary Components*. National Institutes of Health; 2010. Updated November 30, 2019. Accessed July 9, 2025. https://epi.grants.cancer.gov/diet/foodsources/top-food-sources-report-02212020.pdf

100   Revealing trans fats. *FDA Consumer*. 2003;37(5):20–6. Accessed July 19, 2025. https://webharvest.gov/peth04/20041109085957/http://www.fda.gov/fdac/features/2003/503_fats.html

101   US Department of Health and Human Services, US Food and Drug Administration. 21 CFR Parts 161,164,184,186. Food additives permitted for direct addition to food for human consumption; final rule. *Fed Regist*. 2023;88(152):53764–74.

102   Verneque BJF, Machado AM, de Abreu Silva L, Lopes ACS, Duarte CK. Ruminant and industrial trans-fatty acids consumption and cardiometabolic risk markers: a systematic review. *Crit Rev Food Sci Nutr*. 2022;62(8):2050–60.

103   Revealing trans fats. *FDA Consumer*. 2003;37(5):20–6. Accessed July 19, 2025. https://webharvest.gov/peth04/20041109085957/http://www.fda.gov/fdac/features/2003/503_fats.html

104   Fox M. Report recommends limiting trans-fats in diet. *Reuters*. July 10, 2002.

105   National Cancer Institute. *Identification of Top Food Sources of Various Dietary Components*. National Institutes of Health; 2010. Updated November 30, 2019. Accessed July 9, 2025. https://epi.grants.cancer.gov/diet/foodsources/top-food-sources-report-02212020.pdf

106   Guasch-Ferré M, Satija A, Blondin SA, et al. Meta-analysis of randomized controlled trials of red meat consumption in comparison with various comparison diets on cardiovascular risk factors. *Circulation*. 2019;139(15):1828–45. doi:10.1161/CIRCULATIONAHA.118.035225

107   US dietary guidelines remove dietary cholesterol limit. British Lion Eggs. August 1, 2016. Accessed July 8, 2025. https://www.egginfo.co.uk/news/us-dietary-guidelines-remove-dietary-cholesterol-limit

108   US Department of Health and Human Services, US Department of Agriculture. *2015-2020 Dietary Guidelines for Americans*. 8th ed. DietaryGuidelines.gov; 2015.

109   US Department of Health and Human Services, US Department of Agriculture. *2020-2025 Dietary Guidelines for Americans*. 9th ed. DietaryGuidelines.gov; 2020.

110   Grundy SM. Does dietary cholesterol matter? *Curr Atheroscler Rep*. 2016;18(11):68. doi: 10.1007/s11883-016-0615-0

111   De Biase SG, Fernandes SF, Gianini RJ, Duarte JL. Vegetarian diet and cholesterol and triglycerides levels. *Arq Bras Cardiol*. 2007;88(1):35–9. doi: 10.1590/s0066-782x2007000100006

112 Penson PE, Pirro M, Banach M. LDL-C: lower is better for longer—even at low risk. *BMC Med*. 2020;18(1):320. doi: 10.1186/s12916-020-01792-7

113 Kendall CW, Jenkins DJ. A dietary portfolio: maximal reduction of low-density lipoprotein cholesterol with diet. *Curr Atheroscler Rep*. 2004;6(6):492–8. doi: 10.1007/s11883-004-0091-9

114 Chiavaroli L, Nishi SK, Khan TA, et al. Portfolio dietary pattern and cardiovascular disease: a systematic review and meta-analysis of controlled trials. *Prog Cardiovasc Dis*. 2018;61(1):43–53. doi: 10.1016/j.pcad.2018.05.004

115 Jenkins DJ, Kendall CW, Marchie A, et al. Direct comparison of a dietary portfolio of cholesterol-lowering foods with a statin in hypercholesterolemic participants. *Am J Clin Nutr*. 2005;81(2):380–7. doi: 10.1093/ajcn.81.2.380

116 Chiavaroli L, Nishi SK, Khan TA, et al. Portfolio dietary pattern and cardiovascular disease: a systematic review and meta-analysis of controlled trials. *Prog Cardiovasc Dis*. 2018;61(1):43–53. doi: 10.1016/j.pcad.2018.05.004

117 Jenkins DJ, Jones PJ, Lamarche B, et al. Effect of a dietary portfolio of cholesterol-lowering foods given at 2 levels of intensity of dietary advice on serum lipids in hyperlipidemia: a randomized controlled trial. *JAMA*. 2011;306(8):831–9. doi: 10.1001/jama.2011.1202

118 Jenkins DJ, Kendall CW, Faulkner D, et al. A dietary portfolio approach to cholesterol reduction: combined effects of plant sterols, vegetable proteins, and viscous fibers in hypercholesterolemia. *Metabolism*. 2002;51(12):1596–604. doi: 10.1053/meta.2002.35578

119 Benecol. Olive Premium Products Corporation. Accessed July 9, 2025. https://www.benecolusa.com/products

120 Promise, Activ, Light, 35% vegetable oil spread. Prospre. Accessed July 9, 2025. https://www.prospre.io/ingredients/promise-activ-light-35-vegetable-oil-spread-58834

121 Phillips KM, Ruggio DM, Ashraf-Khorassani M. Phytosterol composition of nuts and seeds commonly consumed in the United States. *J Agric Food Chem*. 2005;53(24):9436–45. doi: 10.1021/jf051505h

122 Ryan E, Galvin K, O'Connor TP, Maguire AR, O'Brien NM. Phytosterol, squalene, tocopherol content and fatty acid profile of selected seeds, grains, and legumes. *Plant Foods Hum Nutr*. 2007;62(3):85–91. doi: 10.1007/s11130-007-0046-8

123 Spiller G, ed. *Topics in Dietary Fiber Research*. Plenum Press; 1978.

124 Eaton SB, Eaton SB, Konner MJ. Paleolithic nutrition revisited: a twelve-year retrospective on its nature and implications. *Eur J Clin Nutr*. 1997;51(4):207–16.

125 Agricultural Research Service, United States Department of Agriculture. *Usual Nutrient Intake from Food and Beverages, by Gender and Age, What We Eat in America, NHANES 2015–2018*. United States Department of Agriculture; 2021. Accessed July 9, 2025. https://www.ars.usda.gov/ARSUserFiles/80400530/pdf/usual/Usual_Intake_gender_WWEIA_2015_2018.pdf

126 Eaton SB, Eaton SB, Konner MJ. Paleolithic nutrition revisited: a twelve-year retrospective on its nature and implications. *Eur J Clin Nutr*. 1997;51(4):207–16. doi: 10.1038/sj.ejcn.1600389

127 Jenkins DJ, Kendall CW, Chiavaroli L, et al. The Portfolio Diet: an evidence-based eating plan for lower cholesterol. Canadian Cardiovascular Society. November 2023. Accessed July 9, 2025. https://ccs.ca/wp-content/uploads/2023/11/Portfolio-Infographic-EN_7Nov2023.pdf

128 Jefrei E, Xu M, Moore JB, Thorne JL. Phytosterol and phytostanol-mediated epigenetic changes in cancer and other non-communicable diseases: a systematic review. *Br J Nutr*. 2024;131(6):935–43. doi: 10.1017/S0007114523002532

129 Racette SB, Lin X, Lefevre M, et al. Dose effects of dietary phytosterols on cholesterol metabolism: a controlled feeding study. *Am J Clin Nutr*. 2010;91(1):32–8. doi: 10.3945/ajcn.2009.28070

130 Jones PJH, Shamloo M, MacKay DS, et al. Progress and perspectives in plant sterol and plant stanol research. *Nutr Rev*. 2018;76(10):725–46. doi: 10.1093/nutrit/nuy032

131 Cofán M, Ros E. Use of plant sterol and stanol fortified foods in clinical practice. *Curr Med Chem*. 2019;26(37):6691–703. doi: 10.2174/0929867325666180709114524

132 Vezza T, Canet F, de Marañón AM, Bañuls C, Rocha M, Víctor VM. Phytosterols: nutritional health players in the management of obesity and its related disorders. *Antioxidants*. 2020;9(12):1266. doi: 10.3390/antiox9121266

133 Phillips KM, Ruggio DM, Ashraf-Khorassani M. Phytosterol composition of nuts and seeds commonly consumed in the United States. *J Agric Food Chem*. 2005;53(24):9436–45. doi: 10.1021/jf051505h

134 Del Gobbo LC, Falk MC, Feldman R, Lewis K, Mozaffarian D. Are phytosterols responsible for the low-density lipoprotein-lowering effects of tree nuts?: a systematic review and meta-analysis. *J Am Coll Cardiol*. 2015;65(25):2765–7. doi: 10.1016/j.jacc.2015.03.595

135 Jenkins DJ, Kendall CW, Chiavaroli L, et al. The Portfolio Diet: an evidence-based eating plan for lower cholesterol. Canadian Cardiovascular Society. November 2023. Accessed July 9, 2025. https://ccs.ca/wp-content/uploads/2023/11/Portfolio-Infographic-EN_7Nov2023.pdf

136 Del Gobbo LC, Falk MC, Feldman R, Lewis K, Mozaffarian D. Are phytosterols responsible for the low-density lipoprotein-lowering effects of tree nuts?: a systematic review and meta-analysis. *J Am Coll Cardiol*. 2015;65(25):2765–7. doi: 10.1016/j.jacc.2015.03.595

137 Racette SB, Lin X, Lefevre M, et al. Dose effects of dietary phytosterols on cholesterol metabolism: a controlled feeding study. *Am J Clin Nutr*. 2010;91(1):32–8. doi: 10.3945/ajcn.2009.28070

138 Ras RT, Geleijnse JM, Trautwein EA. LDL-cholesterol-lowering effect of plant sterols and stanols across different dose ranges: a meta-analysis of randomised controlled studies. *Br J Nutr*. 2014;112(2):214–9. doi: 10.1017/S0007114514000750

139 Ference BA, Ginsberg HN, Graham I, et al. Low-density lipoproteins cause atherosclerotic cardiovascular disease. 1. Evidence from genetic, epidemiologic, and clinical studies. A consensus statement from the European Atherosclerosis Society Consensus Panel. *Eur Heart J*. 2017;38(32):2459–72. doi: 10.1093/eurheartj/ehx144

140 Zhang YF, Qiao W, Feng H, et al. Effects of phytosterol supplementation on lipid profiles and apolipoproteins: a meta-analysis of randomized controlled trials. *Medicine*. 2024;103(42):e40020. doi: 10.1097/MD.0000000000040020

141 Lizard G. Phytosterols: to be or not to be toxic; that is the question. *Br J Nutr*. 2008;100(6):1150–1. doi: 10.1017/S0007114508986888

142 Poli A, Marangoni F, Corsini A, et al. Phytosterols, cholesterol control, and cardiovascular disease. *Nutrients*. 2021;13(8):2810. doi: 10.3390/nu13082810

143 Willems JI, Blommaert MA, Trautwein EA. Results from a post-launch monitoring survey on consumer purchases of foods with added phytosterols in five European countries. *Food Chem Toxicol*. 2013;62:48–53. doi: 10.1016/j.fct.2013.08.021

144 Stock J. Focus on lifestyle: EAS Consensus Panel position statement on phytosterol-added foods. *Atherosclerosis*. 2014;234(1):142–5. doi: 10.1016/j.atherosclerosis.2014.01.047

145 Jiang L, Zhao X, Xu J, et al. The protective effect of dietary phytosterols on cancer risk: a systematic meta-analysis. *J Oncol*. 2019;2019:7479518. doi: 10.1155/2019/7479518

146 Balakrishna R, Bjørnerud T, Bemanian M, Aune D, Fadnes LT. Consumption of nuts and seeds and health outcomes including cardiovascular disease, diabetes and metabolic disease, cancer, and mortality: an umbrella review. *Adv Nutr*. 2022;13(6):2136–48. doi: 10.1093/advances/nmac077

147 Balakrishna R, Bjørnerud T, Bemanian M, Aune D, Fadnes LT. Consumption of nuts and seeds and health outcomes including cardiovascular disease, diabetes and metabolic disease, cancer, and mortality: an umbrella review. *Adv Nutr*. 2022;13(6):2136–48. doi: 10.1093/advances/nmac077

148 Jefrei E, Xu M, Moore JB, Thorne JL. Phytosterol and phytostanol-mediated epigenetic changes in cancer and other non-communicable diseases: a systematic review. *Br J Nutr*. 2024;131(6):935–43. doi: 10.1017/S0007114523002532

149 Cancer drug costs for a month of treatment at initial Food and Drug Administration approval. Memorial Sloan Kettering Cancer Center. Accessed July 9, 2025. https://www.mskcc.org/sites/default/files/node/25097/documents/111516-drug-costs-table.pdf

150 Jefrei E, Xu M, Moore JB, Thorne JL. Phytosterol and phytostanol-mediated epigenetic changes in cancer and other non-communicable diseases: a systematic review. *Br J Nutr*. 2024;131(6):935–43. doi: 10.1017/S0007114523002532

151 Fardet A, Morise A, Kalonji E, Margaritis I, Mariotti F. Influence of phytosterol and phytostanol food supplementation on plasma liposoluble vitamins and provitamin A carotenoid levels in humans: an updated review of the evidence. *Crit Rev Food Sci Nutr*. 2017;57(9):1906–21. doi: 10.1080/10408398.2015.1033611

152 Hoekstra J, Fransen HP, van Eijkeren JC, et al. Benefit-risk assessment of plant sterols in margarine: a QALIBRA case study. *Food Chem Toxicol*. 2013;54:35–42. doi: 10.1016/j.fct.2012.08.054

153 Stock J. Focus on lifestyle: EAS Consensus Panel position statement on phytosterol-added foods. *Atherosclerosis*. 2014;234(1):142–5. doi: 10.1016/j.atherosclerosis.2014.01.047

154 Shen M, Yuan L, Zhang J, et al. Phytosterols: physiological functions and potential application. *Foods*. 2024;13(11):1754. doi: 10.3390/foods13111754

155 Feng S, Belwal T, Li L, Limwachiranon J, Liu X, Luo Z. Phytosterols and their derivatives: potential health-promoting uses against lipid metabolism and associated diseases, mechanism, and safety issues. *Compr Rev Food Sci Food Saf*. 2020;19(4):1243–67. doi: 10.1111/1541-4337.12560

156 Turck D, Castenmiller J, De Henauw S, et al. Safety of the extension of use of plant sterol esters as a novel food pursuant to regulation (EU) 2015/2283. *EFSA J.* 2020;18(6):e06135. doi: 10.2903/j.efsa.2020.6135

157 Feng S, Belwal T, Li L, Limwachiranon J, Liu X, Luo Z. Phytosterols and their derivatives: potential health-promoting uses against lipid metabolism and associated diseases, mechanism, and safety issues. *Compr Rev Food Sci Food Saf.* 2020;19(4):1243–67. doi: 10.1111/1541-4337

158 Ratnayake WM, L'Abbé MR, Mueller R, et al. Vegetable oils high in phytosterols make erythrocytes less deformable and shorten the life span of stroke-prone spontaneously hypertensive rats. *J Nutr.* 2000;130(5):1166–78. doi: 10.1093/jn/130.5.1166

159 Moghadasian MH, Nguyen LB, Shefer S, McManus BM, Frohlich JJ. Histologic, hematologic, and biochemical characteristics of apo E-deficient mice: effects of dietary cholesterol and phytosterols. *Lab Invest.* 1999;79(3):355–64. PMID: 10092072

160 Ebine N, Jia X, Demonty I, Wang Y, Jones PJ. Effects of a water-soluble phytostanol ester on plasma cholesterol levels and red blood cell fragility in hamsters. *Lipids.* 2005;40(2):175–80. doi: 10.1007/s11745-005-1373-5

161 de Jong A, Plat J, Mensink RP. Plant sterol or stanol consumption does not affect erythrocyte osmotic fragility in patients on statin treatment. *Eur J Clin Nutr.* 2006;60(8):985–90. doi: 10.1038/sj.ejcn.1602409

162 Windler E, Beil FU, Berthold HK, et al. Phytosterols and cardiovascular risk evaluated against the background of phytosterolemia cases — a German expert panel statement. *Nutrients.* 2023;15(4):828. doi: 10.3390/nu15040828

163 Harcombe Z, Baker JS. Plant sterols lower cholesterol, but increase risk for coronary heart disease. *Online J Biol Sci.* 2014;14(3):167–9. doi: 10.3844/ojbsci.2014.167.169

164 Windler E, Beil FU, Berthold HK, et al. Phytosterols and cardiovascular risk evaluated against the background of phytosterolemia cases — a German expert panel statement. *Nutrients.* 2023;15(4):828. doi: 10.3390/nu15040828

165 Gylling H, Plat J, Turley S, et al; Plant sterols and plant stanols in the management of dyslipidaemia and prevention of cardiovascular disease. *Atherosclerosis.* 2014;232(2):346–60. doi: 10.1016/j.atherosclerosis.2013.11.043

166 Harcombe Z, Baker JS. Plant sterols lower cholesterol, but increase risk for coronary heart disease. *Online J Biol Sci.* 2014;14(3):167–9. doi: 10.3844/ojbsci.2014.167.169

167 Gylling H, Plat J, Turley S, et al; Plant sterols and plant stanols in the management of dyslipidaemia and prevention of cardiovascular disease. *Atherosclerosis.* 2014;232(2):346–60. doi: 10.1016/j.atherosclerosis.2013.11.043

168 Windler E, Beil FU, Berthold HK, et al. Phytosterols and cardiovascular risk evaluated against the background of phytosterolemia cases — a German expert panel statement. *Nutrients.* 2023;15(4):828. doi: 10.3390/nu15040828

169 Jones PJH, Shamloo M, MacKay DS, et al. Progress and perspectives in plant sterol and plant stanol research. *Nutr Rev.* 2018;76(10):725–46. doi: 10.1093/nutrit/nuy032

170 Silbernagel G, Baumgartner I, März W. Cardiovascular safety of plant sterol and stanol consumption. *J AOAC Int.* 2015;98(3):739–41. doi: 10.5740/jaoacint.SGESilbernagel

171. Helgadottir A, Thorleifsson G, Alexandersson KF, et al. Genetic variability in the absorption of dietary sterols affects the risk of coronary artery disease. *Eur Heart J*. 2020;41(28):2618–28. doi: 10.1093/eurheartj/ehaa531

172. Windler E, Beil FU, Berthold HK, et al. Phytosterols and cardiovascular risk evaluated against the background of phytosterolemia cases — a German expert panel statement. *Nutrients*. 2023;15(4):828.

173. Windler E, Beil FU, Berthold HK, et al. Phytosterols and cardiovascular risk evaluated against the background of phytosterolemia cases — a German expert panel statement. *Nutrients*. 2023;15(4):828. doi: 10.3390/nu15040828

174. Stock J. Focus on lifestyle: EAS Consensus Panel position statement on phytosterol-added foods. *Atherosclerosis*. 2014;234(1):142–5. doi: 10.1016/j.atherosclerosis.2014.01.047

175. Hoekstra J, Fransen HP, van Eijkeren JC, et al. Benefit-risk assessment of plant sterols in margarine: a QALIBRA case study. *Food Chem Toxicol*. 2013;54:35–42. doi: 10.1016/j.fct.2012.08.054

176. Willems JI, Blommaert MA, Trautwein EA. Results from a post-launch monitoring survey on consumer purchases of foods with added phytosterols in five European countries. *Food Chem Toxicol*. 2013;62:48–53. doi: 10.1016/j.fct.2013.08.021

177. Gylling H, Plat J, Turley S, et al. Supplementary material for: Plant sterols and plant stanols in the management of dyslipidaemia and prevention of cardiovascular disease. *Atherosclerosis*. 2014;232(2):346–60. doi: 10.1016/j.atherosclerosis.2013.11.043

178. Poli A, Marangoni F, Corsini A, et al. Phytosterols, cholesterol control, and cardiovascular disease. *Nutrients*. 2021;13(8):2810. doi: 10.3390/nu13082810

179. Silverman MG, Ference BA, Im K, et al. Association between lowering LDL-C and cardiovascular risk reduction among different therapeutic interventions: a systematic review and meta-analysis. *JAMA*. 2016;316(12):1289–97. doi: 10.1001/jama.2016.13985

180. Klingel R, Heibges A, Fassbender C. Lipoprotein apheresis results in plaque stabilization and prevention of cardiovascular events: comments on the prospective Pro(a)LiFe study. *Clin Res Cardiol Suppl*. 2015;10(Suppl 1):46–50. doi: 10.1007/s11789-015-0068-y

181. Landray MJ, Haynes R, Hopewell JC, et al. Effects of extended-release niacin with laropiprant in high-risk patients. *N Engl J Med*. 2014;371(3):203–12. doi: 10.1056/NEJMoa1300955

182. Gylling H, Strandberg TE, Kovanen PT, Simonen P. Lowering low-density lipoprotein cholesterol concentration with plant stanol esters to reduce the risk of atherosclerotic cardiovascular disease events at a population level: a critical discussion. *Nutrients*. 2020;12(8):2346. doi: 10.3390/nu12082346

183. Cannon CP, Blazing MA, Giugliano RP, et al. Ezetimibe added to statin therapy after acute coronary syndromes. *N Engl J Med*. 2015;372(25):2387–97. doi: 10.1056/NEJMoa1410489

184. Yang Y, Xia J, Yu T, Wan S, Zhou Y, Sun G. Effects of phytosterols on cardiovascular risk factors: a systematic review and meta-analysis of randomized controlled trials. *Phytother Res*. 2025;39(1):3–24. doi: 10.1002/ptr.8308

185 Clarenbach JJ, Reber M, Lütjohann D, von Bergmann K, Sudhop T. The lipid-lowering effect of ezetimibe in pure vegetarians. *J Lipid Res*. 2006;47(12):2820–4. doi: 10.1194/jlr.P600009-JLR200

186 Malina DM, Fonseca FA, Barbosa SA, et al. Additive effects of plant sterols supplementation in addition to different lipid-lowering regimens. *J Clin Lipidol*. 2015;9(4):542–52. doi: 10.1016/j.jacl.2015.04.003

187 Cofán M, Ros E. Use of plant sterol and stanol fortified foods in clinical practice. *Curr Med Chem*. 2019;26(37):6691–703. doi: 10.2174/0929867325666180709114524

188 Wang T, Ma C, Hu Y, et al. Effects of food formulation on bioavailability of phytosterols: phytosterol structures, delivery carriers, and food matrices. *Food Funct*. 2023;14(12):5465–77. doi: 10.1039/d3fo00566f

189 Demonty I, Ras RT, van der Knaap HC, et al. Continuous dose-response relationship of the LDL-cholesterol-lowering effect of phytosterol intake. *J Nutr*. 2009;139(2):271–84. doi: 10.3945/jn.108.095125

190 Musa-Veloso K, Poon TH, Elliot JA, Chung C. A comparison of the LDL-cholesterol lowering efficacy of plant stanols and plant sterols over a continuous dose range: results of a meta-analysis of randomized, placebo-controlled trials. *Prostaglandins Leukot Essent Fatty Acids*. 2011;85(1):9–28. doi: 10.1016/j.plefa.2011.02.001

191 Plant sterols and stanols in foods and supplements. National Lipid Association. Accessed July 9, 2025. https://www.lipid.org/sites/default/files/plant_sterols_im_food_sterol_supplements.pdf

192 Cofán M, Ros E. Use of plant sterol and stanol fortified foods in clinical practice. *Curr Med Chem*. 2019;26(37):6691–703. doi: 10.2174/0929867325666180709114524

193 Rosin S, Ojansivu I, Kopu A, Keto-Tokoi M, Gylling H. Optimal use of plant stanol ester in the management of hypercholesterolemia. *Cholesterol*. 2015;2015:706970. doi: 10.1155/2015/706970

194 Amir Shaghaghi M, Abumweis SS, Jones PJH. Cholesterol-lowering efficacy of plant sterols/stanols provided in capsule and tablet formats: results of a systematic review and meta-analysis. *J Acad Nutr Diet*. 2013;113(11):1494–503. doi: 10.1016/j.jand.2013.07.006

195 McGowan MP, Proulx S. Nutritional supplements and serum lipids: does anything work? *Curr Atheroscler Rep*. 2009;11(6):470–6. doi: 10.1007/s11883-009-0070-2

196 Weet-Bix: cholesterol lowering. Sanitarium Health Food Company. Accessed July 9, 2025. https://weetbix.com.au/products/weet-bix-added-benefits/Cholesterol-Lowering-440g

197 Plant sterols and stanols in foods and supplements. National Lipid Association. Accessed July 9, 2025. https://www.lipid.org/sites/default/files/plant_sterols_im_food_sterol_supplements.pdf

198 CholestOff Complete softgels. Nature Made. Accessed April 30, 2025. https://www.naturemade.com/products/cholestoff-complete

199 CholestaCare. ProCaps. Accessed April 30, 2025. https://www.procapslabs.com/Products/CholestaCare/301513/

200 Foresterol. designs for health. Accessed April 30, 2025. https://www.designsforhealth.com/products/foresterol

201 ModuChol. Wakunaga of America. Accessed July 9, 2025. https://kyolic.com/product/moduchol/

202 Phytosterols Powder. BulkSupplements.com. Accessed April 30, 2025. https://www.bulksupplements.com/products/phytosterol-beta-sitosterol-powder

203 Plant Sterols. New Roots Herbal. Accessed April 30, 2025. https://newrootsherbal.com/shop/plant-sterols

204 Pouteau EB, Monnard IE, Piguet-Welsch C, Groux MJ, Sagalowicz L, Berger A. Non-esterified plant sterols solubilized in low fat milks inhibit cholesterol absorption — a stable isotope double-blind crossover study. *Eur J Nutr*. 2003;42(3):154–64. doi: 10.1007/s00394-003-0406-6

205 Rondanelli M, Monteferrario F, Faliva MA, Perna S, Antoniello N. Key points for maximum effectiveness and safety for cholesterol-lowering properties of plant sterols and use in the treatment of metabolic syndrome. *J Sci Food Agric*. 2013;93(11):2605–10. doi: 10.1002/jsfa.6174

206 Amir Shaghaghi M, Abumweis SS, Jones PJH. Cholesterol-lowering efficacy of plant sterols/stanols provided in capsule and tablet formats: results of a systematic review and meta-analysis. *J Acad Nutr Diet*. 2013;113(11):1494–503. doi: 10.1016/j.jand.2013.07.006

207 Richelle M, Enslen M, Hager C, et al. Both free and esterified plant sterols reduce cholesterol absorption and the bioavailability of beta-carotene and alpha-tocopherol in normocholesterolemic humans. *Am J Clin Nutr*. 2004;80(1):171–7. doi: 10.1093/ajcn/80.1.171

208 Thomsen AB, Hansen HB, Christiansen C, Green H, Berger A. Effect of free plant sterols in low-fat milk on serum lipid profile in hypercholesterolemic subjects. *Eur J Clin Nutr*. 2004;58(6):860–70. doi: 10.1038/sj.ejcn.1601887

209 Rideout TC. Getting personal: considering variable interindividual responsiveness to dietary lipid-lowering therapies. *Curr Opin Lipidol*. 2011;22(1):37–42. doi: 10.1097/MOL.0b013e3283414e71

210 Rideout TC, Harding SV, Mackay DS. Metabolic and genetic factors modulating subject specific LDL-C responses to plant sterol therapy. *Can J Physiol Pharmacol*. 2012;90(5):509–14. doi: 10.1139/y2012-060

211 Simonen P, Nylund L, Vartiainen E, et al. Heart-healthy diets including phytostanol ester consumption to reduce the risk of atherosclerotic cardiovascular diseases. A clinical review. *Lipids Health Dis*. 2024;23(1):341. doi: 10.1186/s12944-024-02330-7

212 Cicero AFG, Colletti A, Bajraktari G, et al. Lipid lowering nutraceuticals in clinical practice: position paper from an International Lipid Expert Panel. *Arch Med Sci*. 2017;13(5):965–1005. doi: 10.5114/aoms.2017.69326

213 Chen JT, Wesley R, Shamburek RD, Pucino F, Csako G. Meta-analysis of natural therapies for hyperlipidemia: plant sterols and stanols versus policosanol. *Pharmacotherapy*. 2005;25(2):171–83. doi: 10.1592/phco.25.2.171.56942

214 Castaño G, Menéndez R, Más R, et al. Effects of policosanol and lovastatin on lipid profile and lipid peroxidation in patients with dyslipidemia associated with type 2 diabetes mellitus. *Int J Clin Pharmacol Res*. 2002;22(3-4):89–99. PMID: 12837046

215 Chen JT, Wesley R, Shamburek RD, Pucino F, Csako G. Meta-analysis of natural therapies for hyperlipidemia: plant sterols and stanols versus policosanol. *Pharmacotherapy*. 2005;25(2):171–83. doi: 10.1592/phco.25.2.171.56942

216 Kassis AN, Jones PJ. Lack of cholesterol-lowering efficacy of Cuban sugar cane policosanols in hypercholesterolemic persons. *Am J Clin Nutr*. 2006;84(5):1003–8. doi: 10.1093/ajcn/84.5.1003

217 Berthold HK, Unverdorben S, Degenhardt R, Bulitta M, Gouni-Berthold I. Effect of policosanol on lipid levels among patients with hypercholesterolemia or combined hyperlipidemia: a randomized controlled trial. *JAMA*. 2006;295(19):2262–9. doi: 10.1001/jama.295.19.2262

218 Kassis AN, Jones PJ. Lack of cholesterol-lowering efficacy of Cuban sugar cane policosanols in hypercholesterolemic persons. *Am J Clin Nutr*. 2006;84(5):1003–8. doi: 10.1093/ajcn/84.5.1003

219 Marinangeli CP, Jones PJ, Kassis AN, Eskin MN. Policosanols as nutraceuticals: fact or fiction. *Crit Rev Food Sci Nutr*. 2010;50(3):259–67. doi: 10.1080/10408391003626249

220 Kassis AN, Jones PJ. Lack of cholesterol-lowering efficacy of Cuban sugar cane policosanols in hypercholesterolemic persons. *Am J Clin Nutr*. 2006;84(5):1003–8. doi: 10.1093/ajcn/84.5.1003

221 Berthold HK, Unverdorben S, Degenhardt R, Bulitta M, Gouni-Berthold I. Effect of policosanol on lipid levels among patients with hypercholesterolemia or combined hyperlipidemia: a randomized controlled trial. *JAMA*. 2006;295(19):2262–9. doi: 10.1001/jama.295.19.2262

222 Jones PJH, Kassis AN, Marinangeli CPF. Policosanols lose their lustre as cholesterol-lowering agents. *J Funct Foods*. 2009;1(2):236–9. doi: 10.1016/j.jff.2009.01.001

223 Gong J, Qin X, Yuan F, et al. Efficacy and safety of sugarcane policosanol on dyslipidemia: a meta-analysis of randomized controlled trials. *Mol Nutr Food Res*. 2018;62(1). doi: 10.1002/mnfr.201700280

224 McGowan MP, Proulx S. Nutritional supplements and serum lipids: does anything work? *Curr Atheroscler Rep*. 2009;11(6):470–6. doi: 10.1007/s11883-009-0070-2

225 Trogkanis E, Karalexi MA, Sergentanis TN, Kornarou E, Vassilakou T. Safety and efficacy of the consumption of the nutraceutical "red yeast rice extract" for the reduction of hypercholesterolemia in humans: a systematic review and meta-analysis. *Nutrients*. 2024;16(10):1453. doi: 10.3390/nu16101453

226 Sungthong B, Yoothaekool C, Promphamorn S, Phimarn W. Efficacy of red yeast rice extract on myocardial infarction patients with borderline hypercholesterolemia: a meta-analysis of randomized controlled trials. *Sci Rep*. 2020;10(1):2769. doi: 10.1038/s41598-020-59796-5

227 Zhao SP, Lu ZL, Du BM, et al. Xuezhikang, an extract of cholestin, reduces cardiovascular events in type 2 diabetes patients with coronary heart disease: subgroup analysis of patients with type 2 diabetes from China Coronary Secondary Prevention Study (CCSPS). *J Cardiovasc Pharmacol*. 2007;49(2):81–4. doi: 10.1097/FJC.0b013e31802d3a58.

228 Trogkanis E, Karalexi MA, Sergentanis TN, Kornarou E, Vassilakou T. Safety and efficacy of the consumption of the nutraceutical "red yeast rice extract" for the reduction of hypercholesterolemia in humans: a systematic review and meta-analysis. *Nutrients*. 2024;16(10):1453. doi: 10.3390/nu16101453

229 Dujovne CA. Red yeast rice preparations: are they suitable substitutions for statins? *Am J Med*. 2017;130(10):1148–50. doi: 10.1016/j.amjmed.2017.05.013

230 Dujovne CA. Red yeast rice preparations: are they suitable substitutions for statins? *Am J Med*. 2017;130(10):1148–50. doi: 10.1016/j.amjmed.2017.05.013

231 Cohen PA, Avula B, Khan IA. Variability in strength of red yeast rice supplements purchased from mainstream retailers. *Eur J Prev Cardiol*. 2017;24(13):1431–4. doi: 10.1177/2047487317715714

232 Gordon RY, Cooperman T, Obermeyer W, Becker DJ. Marked variability of monacolin levels in commercial red yeast rice products: buyer beware! *Arch Intern Med*. 2010;170(19):1722–7. doi: 10.1001/archinternmed.2010.382

233 Righetti L, Dall'Asta C, Bruni R. Risk assessment of RYR food supplements: perception vs. reality. *Front Nutr*. 2021;8:792529. doi: 10.3389/fnut.2021.792529

234 Gordon RY, Cooperman T, Obermeyer W, Becker DJ. Marked variability of monacolin levels in commercial red yeast rice products: buyer beware! *Arch Intern Med*. 2010;170(19):1722–7. doi: 10.1001/archinternmed.2010.382

235 Backes JM, Hilleman DE. A clinicians guide to recommending common cholesterol-lowering dietary supplements. *Am J Cardiovasc Drugs*. 2024;24(6):719–28. doi: 10.1007/s40256-024-00681-1

236 Backes JM, Hilleman DE. A clinicians guide to recommending common cholesterol-lowering dietary supplements. *Am J Cardiovasc Drugs*. 2024;24(6):719–28. doi: 10.1007/s40256-024-00681-1

237 Miyazaki R, Takahashi Y, Kawamura T, Ueda H, Tsuboi N, Yokoo T. Acute kidney tubular injury after ingestion of red yeast rice supplement. *Clin Kidney J*. 2024;17(6):sfae151. doi: 10.1093/ckj/sfae151

238 Twarużek M, Ałtyn I, Kosicki R. Dietary supplements based on red yeast rice — a source of citrinin? *Toxins*. 2021;13(7):497. doi: 10.3390/toxins13070497

239 Dujovne CA. Red yeast rice preparations: are they suitable substitutions for statins? *Am J Med*. 2017;130(10):1148–50. doi: 10.1016/j.amjmed.2017.05.013

240 Righetti L, Dall'Asta C, Bruni R. Risk assessment of RYR food supplements: perception vs. reality. *Front Nutr*. 2021;8:792529. doi: 10.3389/fnut.2021.792529

241 Righetti L, Dall'Asta C, Bruni R. Risk assessment of RYR food supplements: perception vs. reality. *Front Nutr*. 2021;8:792529. doi: 10.3389/fnut.2021.792529

242 Miyazaki R, Takahashi Y, Kawamura T, Ueda H, Tsuboi N, Yokoo T. Acute kidney tubular injury after ingestion of red yeast rice supplement. *Clin Kidney J*. 2024;17(6):sfae151. doi: 10.1093/ckj/sfae151

243 Shinzawa M, Matsui I, Doi Y, et al. A nationwide questionnaire study evaluated kidney injury associated with Beni-Koji tablets in Japan. *Kidney Int*. 2025;107(3):530–40. doi: 10.1016/j.kint.2024.11.027

244 Murata Y, Hemmi S, Akiya Y, et al. Certain red yeast rice supplements in Japan cause acute tubulointerstitial injury. *Kidney Int Rep*. 2024;9(9):2824–8. doi: 10.1016/j.ekir.2024.06.022

245 Laffin LJ, Nissen SE. Reply: the nuance of studying and prescribing supplements. *J Am Coll Cardiol*. 2023;81(17):e151. doi: 10.1016/j.jacc.2023.02.046

246 Baumgartner S, Bruckert E, Gallo A, Plat J. The position of functional foods and supplements with a serum LDL-C lowering effect in the spectrum ranging from universal to care-related CVD risk management. *Atherosclerosis*. 2020;311:116–23. doi: 10.1016/j.atherosclerosis.2020.07.019

247 Chiavaroli L, Nishi SK, Khan TA, et al. Portfolio dietary pattern and cardiovascular disease: a systematic review and meta-analysis of controlled trials. *Prog Cardiovasc Dis*. 2018;61(1):43–53. doi: 10.1016/j.pcad.2018.05.004

248 Viscous fiber and your cholesterol. National Lipid Association. Accessed May 2, 2025. https://www.lipid.org/sites/default/files/viscous_fiber_and_your_cholesterol.pdf

249 Chiavaroli L, Nishi SK, Khan TA, et al. Portfolio dietary pattern and cardiovascular disease: a systematic review and meta-analysis of controlled trials. *Prog Cardiovasc Dis*. 2018;61(1):43–53. doi: 10.1016/j.pcad.2018.05.004

250 Zhu R, Lei Y, Wang S, et al. Plantago consumption significantly reduces total cholesterol and low-density lipoprotein cholesterol in adults: a systematic review and meta-analysis. *Nutr Res*. 2024;126:123–37. doi: 10.1016/j.nutres.2024.03.013

251 Wei ZH, Wang H, Chen XY, et al. Time- and dose-dependent effect of psyllium on serum lipids in mild-to-moderate hypercholesterolemia: a meta-analysis of controlled clinical trials. *Eur J Clin Nutr*. 2009;63(7):821–7. doi: 10.1038/ejcn.2008.49

252 Arabi SM, Bahrami LS, Rahnama I, Sahebkar A. Impact of synbiotic supplementation on cardiometabolic and anthropometric indices in patients with metabolic syndrome: a systematic review and meta-analysis of randomized controlled trials. *Pharmacol Res*. 2022;176:106061. doi: 10.1016/j.phrs.2022.106061

253 Osadnik T, Goławski M, Lewandowski P, et al. A network meta-analysis on the comparative effect of nutraceuticals on lipid profile in adults. *Pharmacol Res*. 2022;183:106402. doi: 10.1016/j.phrs.2022.106402

254 Osadnik T, Goławski M, Lewandowski P, et al. A network meta-analysis on the comparative effect of nutraceuticals on lipid profile in adults. *Pharmacol Res*. 2022;183:106402. doi: 10.1016/j.phrs.2022.106402

255 Sadeghi-Dehsahraei H, Esmaeili Gouvarchin Ghaleh H, Mirnejad R, Parastouei K. The effect of bergamot (*KoksalGarry*) supplementation on lipid profiles: a systematic review and meta-analysis of randomized controlled trials. *Phytother Res*. 2022;36(12):4409–24. doi: 10.1002/ptr.7647

256 Ferrarese I, Giovanna Lupo M, Rossi I, et al. Bergamot (*Citrus bergamia*) peel extract as new hypocholesterolemic agent modulating PCSK9 expression. *J Funct Foods*. 2023;108:105724. doi: 10.1016/j.jff.2023.105724

257 Liu Y, Zhang S, Jiang T, et al. Mechanistic study of bergamottin-induced inactivation of CYP2C9. *Food Chem Toxicol*. 2021;153:112278. doi: 10.1016/j.fct.2021.112278

258 Finsterer J. Earl Grey tea intoxication. *Lancet*. 2002;359(9316):1484. doi: 10.1016/S0140-6736(02)08436-2

259 Sadeghi-Dehsahraei H, Esmaeili Gouvarchin Ghaleh H, Mirnejad R, Parastouei K. The effect of bergamot (*KoksalGarry*) supplementation on lipid profiles: a systematic review and meta-analysis of randomized controlled trials. *Phytother Res*. 2022;36(12):4409–24. doi: 10.1002/ptr.7647

260 Osadnik T, Goławeski M, Lewandowski P, et al. A network meta-analysis on the comparative effect of nutraceuticals on lipid profile in adults. *Pharmacol Res*. 2022;183:106402. doi: 10.1016/j.phrs.2022.106402

261 Shahinfar H, Bazshahi E, Amini MR, et al. Effects of artichoke leaf extract supplementation or artichoke juice consumption on lipid profile: a systematic review and dose-response meta-analysis of randomized controlled trials. *Phytother Res*. 2021;35(12):6607–23. doi: 10.1002/ptr.7247

262 Schütz K, Muks E, Carle R, Schieber A. Quantitative determination of phenolic compounds in artichoke-based dietary supplements and pharmaceuticals by high-performance liquid chromatography. *J Agric Food Chem*. 2006;54(23):8812–7. doi: 10.1021/jf062009b

263 Mena-García A, Ruiz-Matute AI, Soria AC, Sanz ML. A multi-analytical strategy for evaluation of quality and authenticity of artichoke food supplements for overweight control. *J Chromatogr A*. 2021;1647:462102. doi: 10.1016/j.chroma.2021.462102

264 Santos HO, Bueno AA, Mota JF. The effect of artichoke on lipid profile: a review of possible mechanisms of action. *Pharmacol Res*. 2018;137:170–8. doi: 10.1016/j.phrs.2018.10.007

265 Osadnik T, Goławeski M, Lewandowski P, et al. A network meta-analysis on the comparative effect of nutraceuticals on lipid profile in adults. *Pharmacol Res*. 2022;183:106402. doi: 10.1016/j.phrs.2022.106402

266 Blais JE, Huang X, Zhao JV. Overall and sex-specific effect of berberine for the treatment of dyslipidemia in adults: a systematic review and meta-analysis of randomized placebo-controlled trials. *Drugs*. 2023;83(5):403–27. doi: 10.1007/s40265-023-01841-4

267 Blais JE, Huang X, Zhao JV. Overall and sex-specific effect of berberine for the treatment of dyslipidemia in adults: a systematic review and meta-analysis of randomized placebo-controlled trials. *Drugs*. 2023;83(5):403–27. doi: 10.1007/s40265-023-01841-4

268 Fan J, Liu X, Li Y, et al. Quality problems of clinical trials in China: evidence from quality related studies. *Trials*. 2022;23(1):343. doi: 10.1186/s13063-022-06281-1

269 China's medical research integrity questioned. *Lancet*. 2015;385(9976):1365. doi: 10.1016/S0140-6736(15)60700-0

270 Woodhead M. 80% of China's clinical trial data are fraudulent, investigation finds. *BMJ*. 2016;355:i5396. doi: 10.1136/bmj.i5396

271 Cyranoski D. China cracks down on fake data in drug trials. *Nature*. 2017;545(7654):275. doi: 10.1038/nature.2017.21977

272 Blais JE, Huang X, Zhao JV. Overall and sex-specific effect of berberine for the treatment of dyslipidemia in adults: a systematic review and meta-analysis of randomized placebo-controlled trials. *Drugs*. 2023;83(5):403–27. doi: 10.1007/s40265-023-01841-4

273 Funk RS, Singh RK, Winefield RD, et al. Variability in potency among commercial preparations of berberine. *J Diet Suppl*. 2018;15(3):343–51. doi: 10.1080/19390211.2017.1347227

274 Danoun S, Balayssac S, Gilard V, Martino R, Malet-Martino M. Quality evaluation of berberine food supplements with high-field and compact ¹H NMR spectrometers. *J Pharm Biomed Anal*. 2023;223:115161. doi: 10.1016/j.jpba.2022.115161

275 NOW's testing results of berberine products: December 2023. *Now Foods*. December 2023. Accessed July 9, 2025. https://www.nowfoods.com/healthy-living/articles/nows-testing-results-berberine-products-december-2023

276 Bonnichsen M, Stoklosa T, Bowen D, Majumdar A. Safety first, a harmful interaction between rivaroxaban and berberine. *Intern Med J*. 2022;52(5):887–8. doi: 10.1111/imj.15774

277 Li Z, Wang Y, Xu Q, et al. Berberine and health outcomes: an umbrella review. *Phytother Res*. 2023;37(5):2051–66. doi: 10.1002/ptr.7806

278 Yue SJ, Liu J, Wang WX, et al. Berberine treatment-emergent mild diarrhea associated with gut microbiota dysbiosis. *Biomed Pharmacother*. 2019;116:109002. doi: 10.1016/j.biopha.2019.109002

279 Lan J, Zhao Y, Dong F, et al. Meta-analysis of the effect and safety of berberine in the treatment of type 2 diabetes mellitus, hyperlipemia and hypertension. *J Ethnopharmacol*. 2015;161:69–81. doi: 10.1016/j.jep.2014.09.049

280 Imenshahidi M, Hosseinzadeh H. Berberine and barberry (*Berberis vulgaris*): a clinical review. *Phytother Res*. 2019;33(3):504–23. doi: 10.1002/ptr.6252

281 Shidfar F, Ebrahimi SS, Hosseini S, Heydari I, Shidfar S, Hajhassani G. The effects of *Berberis vulgaris* fruit extract on serum lipoproteins, apoB, apoA-I, homocysteine, glycemic control and total antioxidant capacity in type 2 diabetic patients. *Iran J Pharm Res*. 2012;11(2):643–52. PMID: 24250489

282 Blais JE, Huang X, Zhao JV. Overall and sex-specific effect of berberine for the treatment of dyslipidemia in adults: a systematic review and meta-analysis of randomized placebo-controlled trials. *Drugs*. 2023;83(5):403–27. doi: 10.1007/s40265-023-01841-4

283 Emamat H, Zahedmehr A, Asadian S, Nasrollahzadeh J. The effect of barberry (*Berberis integerrima*) on lipid profile and systemic inflammation in subjects with cardiovascular risk factors: a randomized controlled trial. *BMC Complement Med Ther*. 2022;22(1):59. doi: 10.1186/s12906-022-03539-8

284 Laffin LJ, Bruemmer D, Garcia M, et al. Comparative effects of low-dose rosuvastatin, placebo, and dietary supplements on lipids and inflammatory biomarkers. *J Am Coll Cardiol*. 2023;81(1):1–12. doi: 10.1016/j.jacc.2022.10.013

285 Laffin LJ, Bruemmer D, Garcia M, et al. Comparative effects of low-dose rosuvastatin, placebo, and dietary supplements on lipids and inflammatory biomarkers. *J Am Coll Cardiol*. 2023;81(1):1–12. doi: 10.1016/j.jacc.2022.10.013

286 Laffin LJ, Bruemmer D, Nissen SE. Are dietary supplements beneficial in lowering cholesterol? SPORT reflections and the path forward. *Eur Heart J*. 2023;44(8):638–40. doi: 10.1093/eurheartj/ehac729

287 Maki KC, Dicklin MR. Caution against rejecting all dietary supplements for LDL cholesterol reduction. *J Am Coll Cardiol*. 2023;81(1):13–5. doi: 10.1016/j.jacc.2022.11.004

288 Laffin LJ, Bruemmer D, Nissen SE. Are dietary supplements beneficial in lowering cholesterol? SPORT reflections and the path forward. *Eur Heart J.* 2023;44(8):638–40. doi: 10.1093/eurheartj/ehac729

289 Laffin LJ, Bruemmer D, Garcia M, et al. Comparative effects of low-dose rosuvastatin, placebo, and dietary supplements on lipids and inflammatory biomarkers. *J Am Coll Cardiol.* 2023;81(1):1–12. doi: 10.1016/j.jacc.2022.10.013

290 Full year and Q4 2024 results. AstraZeneca. February 6, 2025. Accessed July 10, 2025. https://www.astrazeneca.com/media-centre/press-releases/2025/full-year-and-q4-2024-results.html

291 Red yeast rice. Arazo Nutrition. Accessed May 5, 2025. https://arazonutrition.com/products/red-yeast-rice

292 Laffin LJ, Bruemmer D, Garcia M, et al. Comparative effects of low-dose rosuvastatin, placebo, and dietary supplements on lipids and inflammatory biomarkers. *J Am Coll Cardiol.* 2023;81(1):1–12. doi: 10.1016/j.jacc.2022.10.013

293 Cooperman T. Red yeast rice supplements review. ConsumerLab.com. May 19, 2022. Updated April 28, 2025. Accessed July 10, 2025. https://www.consumerlab.com/reviews/red-yeast-rice-supplements-review/red-yeast-rice/

294 CholestOff Plus softgels. Nature Made. Accessed July 10, 2025. https://www.naturemade.com/products/cholestoff-plus?variant=17763142729799

295 Mitchell J, Storozynsky E, Lopez AM. The nuance of studying and prescribing supplements. *J Am Coll Cardiol.* 2023;81(17):e149. doi: 10.1016/j.jacc.2023.01.048

296 Rosin S, Ojansivu I, Kopu A, Keto-Tokoi M, Gylling H. Optimal use of plant stanol ester in the management of hypercholesterolemia. *Cholesterol.* 2015;2015:706970. doi: 10.1155/2015/706970

297 Laffin LJ, Bruemmer D, Garcia M, et al. Comparative effects of low-dose rosuvastatin, placebo, and dietary supplements on lipids and inflammatory biomarkers. *J Am Coll Cardiol.* 2023;81(1):1–12. doi: 10.1016/j.jacc.2022.10.013

298 CholestOff Plus softgels. Nature Made. Accessed July 10, 2025. https://www.naturemade.com/products/cholestoff-plus?variant=17763142729799

299 Unhapipatpong C, Julanon N, Shantavasinkul PC, Polruang N, Numthavaj P, Thakkinstian A. An umbrella review of systematic reviews and meta-analyses of randomized controlled trials investigating the effect of curcumin supplementation on lipid profiles. *Nutr Rev.* 2025:nuaf012. doi: 10.1093/nutrit/nuaf012

300 Laffin LJ, Bruemmer D, Garcia M, et al. Comparative effects of low-dose rosuvastatin, placebo, and dietary supplements on lipids and inflammatory biomarkers. *J Am Coll Cardiol.* 2023;81(1):1–12. doi: 10.1016/j.jacc.2022.10.013

301 Kwak JS, Kim JY, Paek Jeet al. Garlic powder intake and cardiovascular risk factors: a meta-analysis of randomized controlled clinical trials. *Nutr Res Pract.* 2014;8(6):644–54. doi: 10.4162/nrp.2014.8.6.644

302 Garlique healthy cholesterol formula. Garlique. Accessed July 10, 2025. https://garlique.com/products/healthy-cholesterol-formula/

303 Organic Ceylon cinnamon, 1200 mg. Nutriflair. Accessed July 10, 2025. https://nutriflair.com/products/organic-ceylon-cinnamon-1200mg-per-serving-120-capsules

304 Maierean SM, Serban MC, Sahebkar A, et al. The effects of cinnamon supplementation on blood lipid concentrations: a systematic review and meta-analysis. *J Clin Lipidol.* 2017;11(6):1393–406. doi: 10.1016/j.jacl.2017.08.004

305 Eslick GD, Howe PR, Smith C, Priest R, Bensoussan A. Benefits of fish oil supplementation in hyperlipidemia: a systematic review and meta-analysis. *Int J Cardiol.* 2009;136(1):4–16. doi: 10.1016/j.ijcard.2008.03.092

306 Laffin LJ, Bruemmer D, Garcia M, et al. Comparative effects of low-dose rosuvastatin, placebo, and dietary supplements on lipids and inflammatory biomarkers. *J Am Coll Cardiol.* 2023;81(1):1–12. doi: 10.1016/j.jacc.2022.10.013

307 Grant JK, Dangl M, Ndumele CE, Michos ED, Martin SS. A historical, evidence-based, and narrative review on commonly used dietary supplements in lipid-lowering. *J Lipid Res.* 2024;65(2):100493. doi: 10.1016/j.jlr.2023.100493

308 Trumbo PR, Shimakawa T. Tolerable upper intake levels for trans fat, saturated fat, and cholesterol. *Nutr Rev.* 2011;69(5):270–8. doi: 10.1111/j.1753-4887.2011.00389.x

309 Jakše B, Jakše B, Pinter S, et al. Dietary intakes and cardiovascular health of healthy adults in short-, medium-, and long-term whole-food plant-based lifestyle program. *Nutrients.* 2019;12(1):55. doi: 10.3390/nu12010055

310 De Biase SG, Fernandes SF, Gianini RJ, Duarte JL. Vegetarian diet and cholesterol and triglycerides levels. *Arq Bras Cardiol.* 2007;88(1):35–9. doi: 10.1590/s0066-782x2007000100006

311 Harland JI. Food combinations for cholesterol lowering. *Nutr Res Rev.* 2012;25(2):249–66. doi: 10.1017/S0954422412000170

312 Penson PE, Pirro M, Banach M. LDL-C: lower is better for longer—even at low risk. *BMC Med.* 2020;18(1):320. doi: 10.1186/s12916-020-01792-7

313 Jenkins DJ, Kendall CW, Chiavaroli L, et al. The Portfolio Diet: an evidence-based eating plan for lower cholesterol. Canadian Cardiovascular Society. November 2023. Accessed April 29, 2025. https://ccs.ca/wp-content/uploads/2023/11/Portfolio-Infographic-EN_7Nov2023.pdf

314 Jenkins DJ, Kendall CW, Chiavaroli L, et al. The Portfolio Diet: an evidence-based eating plan for lower cholesterol. Canadian Cardiovascular Society. November 2023. Accessed April 29, 2025. https://ccs.ca/wp-content/uploads/2023/11/Portfolio-Infographic-EN_7Nov2023.pdf

315 Martínez-Ortega IA, Mesas AE, Bizzozero-Peroni B, et al. Can different types of tree nuts and peanuts induce varied effects on specific blood lipid parameters? A systematic review and network meta-analysis. *Crit Rev Food Sci Nutr.* 2025;65(8):1538–52. doi: 10.1080/10408398.2023.2296559

316 Martínez-Ortega IA, Mesas AE, Bizzozero-Peroni B, et al. Supplementary material for: Can different types of tree nuts and peanuts induce varied effects on specific blood lipid parameters? A systematic review and network meta-analysis. *Crit Rev Food Sci Nutr.* 2025;65(8):1538–52. doi: 10.1080/10408398.2023.2296559

317 Colpo E, Vilanova CD, Brenner Reetz LG, et al. A single consumption of high amounts of the Brazil nuts improves lipid profile of healthy volunteers. *J Nutr Metab.* 2013;2013:653185. doi: 10.1155/2013/653185

318 Mazokopakis EE, Liontiris MI. Commentary: health concerns of Brazil nut consumption. *J Altern Complement Med.* 2018;24(1):3–6. doi: 10.1089/acm.2017.0159

319 Duarte GBS, Reis BZ, Rogero MM, et al. Consumption of Brazil nuts with high selenium levels increased inflammation biomarkers in obese women: a randomized controlled trial. *Nutrition*. 2019;63-64:162–8. doi: 10.1016/j.nut.2019.02.009

320 Colpo E, Carlos Dalton DAV, Luiz Gustavo BR, et al. Brazilian nut consumption by healthy volunteers improves inflammatory parameters. *Nutrition*. 2014;30(4):459–65. doi: 10.1016/j.nut.2013.10.005

321 Jenkins DJ, Kendall CW, Chiavaroli L, et al. The Portfolio Diet: an evidence-based eating plan for lower cholesterol. Canadian Cardiovascular Society. November 2023. Accessed April 29, 2025. https://ccs.ca/wp-content/uploads/2023/11/Portfolio-Infographic-EN_7Nov2023.pdf

322 Lee M, Sorn SR, Park Y, Park HK. Anthocyanin rich-black soybean testa improved visceral fat and plasma lipid profiles in overweight/obese Korean adults: a randomized controlled trial. *J Med Food*. 2016;19(11):995–1003. doi: 10.1089/jmf.2016.3762

323 Black soybeans, organic, 15 oz. Eden Foods. Accessed July 10, 2025. https://store.edenfoods.com/black-soybeans-organic-15-oz

324 Jenkins DJ, Kendall CW, Chiavaroli L, et al. The Portfolio Diet: an evidence-based eating plan for lower cholesterol. Canadian Cardiovascular Society. November 2023. Accessed April 29, 2025. https://ccs.ca/wp-content/uploads/2023/11/Portfolio-Infographic-EN_7Nov2023.pdf

325 Jenkins DJ, Kendall CW, Chiavaroli L, et al. The Portfolio Diet: an evidence-based eating plan for lower cholesterol. Canadian Cardiovascular Society. November 2023. Accessed April 29, 2025. https://ccs.ca/wp-content/uploads/2023/11/Portfolio-Infographic-EN_7Nov2023.pdf

326 Rad SZK, Rameshrad M, Hosseinzadeh H. Toxicology effects of *Berberis vulgaris* (barberry) and its active constituent, berberine: a review. *Iran J Basic Med Sci*. 2017;20(5):516–29. doi:10.22038/IJBMS.2017.8676

327 Peterson JM, Montgomery S, Haddad E, Kearney L, Tonstad S. Effect of consumption of dried California mission figs on lipid concentrations. *Ann Nutr Metab*. 2011;58(3):232–8. doi: 10.1159/000330112

328 Sullivan VK, Petersen KS, Kris-Etherton PM. Dried fruit consumption and cardiometabolic health: a randomised crossover trial. *Br J Nutr*. 2020;124(9):912–21. doi: 10.1017/S0007114520002007

329 Heydarian A, Tahvilian N, Asbaghi O, Cheshmeh S, Nadery M, Aryaeian N. The effects of plum products consumption on lipid profile in adults: a systematic review and dose-response meta-analysis. *Food Sci Nutr*. 2024;12(5):3080–96. doi: 10.1002/fsn3.4000

330 Damani JJ, Rogers CJ, Lee H, et al. Effects of prune (dried plum) supplementation on cardiometabolic health in postmenopausal women: an ancillary analysis of a 12-month randomized controlled trial, The Prune Study. *J Nutr*. 2024;154(5):1604–18. doi: 10.1016/j.tjnut.2024.03.012

331 Chai SC, Hooshmand S, Saadat RL, Payton ME, Brummel-Smith K, Arjmandi BH. Daily apple versus dried plum: impact on cardiovascular disease risk factors in postmenopausal women. *J Acad Nutr Diet*. 2012;112(8):1158–68. doi: 10.1016/j.jand.2012.05.005

332 Hadi A, Askarpour M, Salamat S, Ghaedi E, Symonds ME, Miraghajani M. Effect of flaxseed supplementation on lipid profile: an updated systematic review and dose-response meta-analysis of sixty-two randomized controlled trials. *Pharmacol Res*. 2020;152:104622. doi: 10.1016/j.phrs.2019.104622

333 Mandaşescu S, Mocanu V, Dăscalița AM, et al. Flaxseed supplementation in hyperlipidemic patients. *Rev Med Chir Soc Med Nat Iasi*. 2005;109(3):502–6. PMID: 16607740

334 Acampado LRT, Chiu HHC, Larrazabal RB Jr, Arcellana AES, Añonuevo-Cruz MCS. The efficacy and safety of *Emblica officinalis* aqueous fruit extract among adult patients with dyslipidemia: a systematic review and meta-analysis. *Acta Med Philipp*. 2023;57(5):90–5. doi: 10.47895/amp.vi0.5047

335 Akhtar MS, Ramzan A, Ali A, Ahmad M. Effect of amla fruit (*Emblica officinalis Gaertn*.) on blood glucose and lipid profile of normal subjects and type 2 diabetic patients. *Int J Food Sci Nutr*. 2011;62(6):609–16. doi: 10.3109/09637486.2011.560565

336 Bahari H, Taheri S, Namkhah Z, Barghchi H, Arzhang P, Nattagh-Eshtivani E. Effects of sumac supplementation on lipid profile: a systematic review and meta-analysis of randomized controlled trials. *Phytother Res*. 2024;38(1):241–52. doi: 10.1002/ptr.8046

337 Rouhi-Boroujeni H, Mosharrar S, Gharipour M, Asadi-Samani M, Rouhi-Boroujeni H. Anti-hyperlipidemic effects of sumac (*Rhus coriaria L*.): can sumac strengthen anti-hyperlipidemic effect of statins? *Pharm Lett*. 2016;8(3):143–7 ISSN: 0975-5071.

338 Bastiaan-Net S, Reitsma M, Cordewener JHG, et al. IgE cross-reactivity of cashew nut allergens. *Int Arch Allergy Immunol*. 2019;178(1):19–32. doi: 10.1159/000493100

339 Rounagh M, Musazadeh V, Hosseininejad-Mohebati A, et al. Effects of *Nigella sativa* supplementation on lipid profiles in adults: an updated systematic review and meta-analysis of randomized controlled trials. *Clin Nutr ESPEN*. 2024;61:168–80. doi: 10.1016/j.clnesp.2024.03.020

340 Alamri E. Comparison of the effect of *Nigella sativa* seeds and powder on lipid profile in Saudi Arabian adults. *Proc Nutr Soc*. 2019;78(OCE1):E12. doi: 10.1017/S0029665119000168

341 Hallajzadeh J, Milajerdi A, Mobini M, et al. Effects of *Nigella sativa* on glycemic control, lipid profiles, and biomarkers of inflammatory and oxidative stress: a systematic review and meta-analysis of randomized controlled clinical trials. *Phytother Res*. 2020;34(10):2586–608. doi: 10.1002/ptr.6708

342 Kwak JS, Kim JY, Paek JE, et al. Garlic powder intake and cardiovascular risk factors: a meta-analysis of randomized controlled clinical trials. *Nutr Res Pract*. 2014;8(6):644–54. doi: 10.4162/nrp.2014.8.6.644

343 Heshmat-Ghahdarijani K, Mashayekhiasl N, Amerizadeh A, Teimouri Jervekani Z, Sadeghi M. Effect of fenugreek consumption on serum lipid profile: a systematic review and meta-analysis. *Phytother Res*. 2020;34(9):2230–45. doi: 10.1002/ptr.6690

344 Kumar K, Kumar S, Datta A, Bandyopadhyay A. Effect of fenugreek seeds on glycemia and dyslipidemia in patients with type 2 diabetes mellitus. *Int J Med Sci Public Health*. 2015;4(7):997. doi: 10.5455/ijmsph.2015.11032015202

345 Shahsavari K, Shams Ardekani MR, Khanavi M, Jamialahmadi T, Iranshahi M, Hasanpour M. Effects of Melissa officinalis (lemon balm) consumption on serum lipid profile: a meta-analysis of randomized controlled trials. *BMC Complement Med Ther*. 2024;24(1):146. doi: 10.1186/s12906-024-04442-0

346 Jandaghi P, Noroozi M, Ardalani H, Alipour M. Lemon balm: a promising herbal therapy for patients with borderline hyperlipidemia — a randomized double-blind placebo-controlled clinical trial. *Complement Ther Med*. 2016;26:136–40. doi: 10.1016/j.ctim.2016.03.012

347 Kheirkhah J, Ghorbani Z, Salari A, et al. Melissa officinalis tea favourably affects the frequency of premature ventricular beats and cardiometabolic profile among patients with premature ventricular contraction: a randomised open-label controlled trial. *Int J Clin Pract*. 2021;75(10):e14644. doi: 10.1111/ijcp.14644

348 Ulbricht C, Brendler T, Gruenwald J, et al. Lemon balm (*Melissa officinalis L.*): an evidence-based systematic review by the Natural Standard Research Collaboration. *J Herb Pharmacother*. 2005;5(4):71–114. PMID: 16635970

349 Nikaein F, Babajafari S, Mazloomi SM, Zibaeenezhad M, Zargaran A. The effects of *Satureja hortensis L.* dried leaves on serum sugar, lipid profiles, hs-CRP, and blood pressure in metabolic syndrome patients: a double-blind randomized clinical trial. *Iran Red Crescent Med J*. 2016;19(1). doi: 10.5812/ircmj.34931

350 Dattilo AM, Kris-Etherton PM. Effects of weight reduction on blood lipids and lipoproteins: a meta-analysis. *Am J Clin Nutr*. 1992;56(2):320–8. doi: 10.1093/ajcn/56.2.320

351 Luo Y, Awoyemi OS, Naidu R, Fang C. Detection of microplastics and nanoplastics released from a kitchen blender using Raman imaging. *J Hazard Mater*. 2023;453:131403. doi: 10.1016/j.jhazmat.2023.131403

352 PubMed search for microplastics or nanoplastics. National Library of Medicine. Accessed May 8, 2025. https://pubmed.ncbi.nlm.nih.gov/?term=microplastics+OR+nanoplastics

353 Wichitsranoi J, Weerapreeyakul N, Boonsiri P, et al. Antihypertensive and antioxidant effects of dietary black sesame meal in pre-hypertensive humans. *Nutr J*. 2011;10:82. doi: 10.1186/1475-2891-10-82

354 Phytosterols powder. BulkSupplements.com. Accessed April 30, 2025. https://www.bulksupplements.com/products/phytosterol-beta-sitosterol-powder

355 Plant sterols. New Roots Herbal. Accessed April 30, 2025. https://newrootsherbal.com/shop/plant-sterols

356 Matyori A, Brown CP, Ali A, Sherbeny F. Statins utilization trends and expenditures in the U.S. before and after the implementation of the 2013 ACC/AHA guidelines. *Saudi Pharm J*. 2023;31(6):795–800. doi: 10.1016/j.jsps.2023.04.002

INDEX

A

American College of Cardiology 3, 15, 35
American Heart Association 3, 4, 15
amla 42, 50, 51
apples 31, 40, 45, 52
artichoke hearts 33, 40, 48
artichoke leaf extracts 33, 40
atorvastatin 12, 13

B

barberries 33, 34, 35, 37, 40, 45, 48, 51
barley 18, 31, 40
beans 18, 39, 40, 45, 49
bempedoic acid 12
berberine 33, 34, 36, 37, 40
bergamot 32, 36, 45, 48, 50, 52
black cumin 42, 51
black sesame seeds 46, 48
black soybeans 39, 45, 51
brazil nuts 38, 45, 51

C

cinnamon 35, 36, 37
citrinin 30
coronary calcium scan 4
corporate determinants of health.
    See commercial determinants of health
Crestor. *See* rosuvastatin
Curcumin. *See* turmeric

D

Daily Dozen 38, 39, 40, 41, 42, 43, 45, 46, 47
dairy 10, 15, 16, 17, 19, 37, 45
DHA 45, 52
diabetes 3, 7
dietary cholesterol 15, 17, 20, 26, 37, 45
Dietary Guidelines 17

E

edible film 50, 52
eggplant 18, 31, 40
eggs 15, 17, 19, 37, 45
Endo, Akira 12
ezetimibe 12

F

Family Heart Foundation 53
fatigue 9
fenugreek 42
fish oil 36, 37
flaxseed 10, 41, 47

G

garlic 35, 36, 37, 42, 51
glucagon-like peptide-1. *See* GLP-1

I

inclisiran 12
Indian gooseberry. *See* amla
iodine 45, 48, 50

K

kelp 48, 50
kidney dysfunction 8

L

leg cramps. *See* quinine
legumes 18, 19, 20, 39
lemon balm 43
Lipitor. *See* atorvastatin
liver dysfunction 8
lovastatin 29, 30
Lyon Diet Heart Study 10

M

meat 10, 15, 16, 17, 19, 37, 45
Mediterranean-style diet 10
Metamucil 31, 47
microplastics 47
Mounjaro. *See* tirzepatide
muscle pain (statin-induced) 8, 9, 15
mushrooms 46, 51

N

niacin 25
nigella seeds. *See* black cumin
nocebo effect 9
nuts 18, 21, 38

O

oats 18, 31, 40
okra 18, 31, 40
Ornish, Dean 10
oxidation products 23
Ozempic. *See* semaglutide

P

PCSK9 inhibitors 12
phytosterolemia 24
plant-based diet 10, 16, 17, 18, 20
plant protein 18
plant sterols 18, 19, 21, 23, 26, 27
policosanol 28, 29
Portfolio Diet 15, 17, 18, 19, 21, 31, 37, 38, 39, 40, 46
Portfolio Plus Powder 46, 48, 49, 51, 52
primary prevention 3, 6, 7, 8, 13, 15, 37
processed foods 16, 37, 45
prunes 40
psyllium 31, 36, 40, 45, 47, 49, 50

R

red blood cell fragility 24
red yeast rice 29, 30, 31, 35, 36
risk calculators 4
rosuvastatin 12, 13, 35, 36

S

saturated fat 12, 15, 17, 18, 37, 45
savory 43, 51
secondary prevention 7, 8
side effects 2, 7, 8, 15
SPORT study 35
statins 2, 3, 4, 5, 6, 7, 8, 9, 11, 12, 15, 18, 25, 29, 37
stroke 3, 7, 8, 48
strokes 1, 7, 8
sumac 42, 48, 49, 50, 52
supplements 19, 27, 28, 29, 30, 31, 32, 33, 34, 35, 36, 37, 40, 45, 48, 54

T

taurine 46, 48, 50, 52
ten-year risk 3, 4, 25, 52
tonic water. *See* quinine
trans fat 15, 16, 37, 45
turmeric 35, 36, 37, 42, 51, 52

U

u-prevent.com 4

V

viscous fiber 18
vitamin B12 45, 49, 50, 52
vitamin D 45, 52

W

walnuts 10, 38
Wegovy. *See* semaglutide
weight loss 46
wheat germ 19, 46, 47, 49

Z

Zepbound. *See* tirzepatide